Old But Still Moving

Staying active while aging, despite life's curveballs
Richard King

To Karen, who has been with me through thick and thin on all our aging adventures.

This book offers health, fitness and nutritional information and is designed for educational purposes only. You should not rely on this information as a substitute for, professional medical advice, diagnosis, or treatment.

<u>**Table of Contents**</u>

August 13th, 2017

I'm in El Camino hospital two days after having major
surgery. I had a heart valve replaced, and my surgeon did a
procedure to fix atrial fibrillation (afib). My sternum was cut
completely in half, and is now held back together with high-
tech bailing wire so it can heal. Under the circumstances, I am
feeling pretty good about how I've been able to get up and
about walking the corridors. But then the physical therapist
takes me to a set of stairs. After going slowly up one flight, I
am on the landing gasping for breath. She says "don't worry,
that's normal". It strikes me: wow, what happened to climbing
up steep hills fast on my bike or on hikes? This is going to be a
long and challenging rehab. Oh, well, I've bounced back from
square one before…

Introduction

There is an old saying "age is a case of mind over matter. If you don't mind, it don't matter". I don't mind the old part, but I do mind the increasing loss of mobility and fitness that have long been thought to be "inevitable" consequences of aging. So I want to describe my attempt to fight them off as I age- as I write this I am 65 and change. I have been active all my life, but I've also had to about roll with the punches, like being told I should no longer run because I had arthritis in my hips. And bouncing back with physical rehab multiple times due to major surgeries- both hips replaced due to defects that led to premature arthritis, and a heart valve replaced due to a genetic defect. This is my story of how I have tried to stay active and healthy as I age, while recovering from the challenges thrown at me.

I also give advice based on what I have learned over the years on physical and mental training as well as diet. There is a lot of confusing and conflicting information on these topics. I am an engineer and comfortable wading through scientific literature, and have tried to come up with an efficient solution to the problem of aging gracefully. Notice I said "tried to", I certainly do not claim to have achieved perfection. There are actually four pillars of longevity, in my opinion. Staying active is one of them, healthy eating is the second, and the others are social support and stress management. I'll give my advice on what I have learned about each of these and what has worked well for me.

Chapter 1 is the fascinating story (at least to me) of my staying active in adulthood, and now "in my later years". One major takeaway from my story was that I have been fortunate to find a way to make physical activities fun. On the couple of occasions where that was temporarily not true, I found what it is like for everyone for whom exercise is a chore that is necessary to stay healthy. I vastly prefer it to be fun. So in chapter 2, I give tips on how to achieve that. Chapter 3 gives activity suggestions for moving throughout the day, aerobic exercise, resistance training, and higher intensity exercise. I switch gears to healthy eating in chapter 4, starting with describing my efforts to eat healthy and avoid middle age spread over the years. The third and fourth aspects, social support and stress management, are covered in chapter 5. Then, in the appendix, I give a lot of background information and cover some miscellaneous topics. Basically anything I thought was too detailed and would make the main part of the book too long-winded got placed there. Hopefully it won't give you appendicitis, something one of my grad school professors claimed about my writing. I wish you a lifetime of good health, enjoyable activity, enjoyable eating without cravings, good support from family and friends, and a strong purpose in life.

Chapter 1. My Adventures in Trying to Age Gracefully

Growing up Active

I was born in 1953 and raised by a single Mom, along with my brother Bill who is 3 ½ years older. My grandma also lived with us. My father had divorced my mother when I was 2. While we did not grow up in the lap of luxury, my Mom did a good job providing for us on a secretary's salary (later as an administrative assistant). My uncle Al and Aunt Martha (nicknamed Aunt Motz), lived a few miles away with my cousins Al and Bob. Al was my age, and Bob about a year and a half younger. They were joined when I was 10 by cousin Scott.

We hung out with their family so much that my cousins were more like brothers to me, Uncle Al was a father figure, and Aunt Motz was like a second Mom. I was very active as a child growing up in central New Jersey, about 30 miles south of New York City. This was suburbia, but at that time it was right on the fringe of the urban sprawl. Just north of us was a lot of heavy industry including major ports and oil refineries, while just south was dairy farm country and thousands of acres of undeveloped land we called "the woods". My brother and cousins and I would disappear into the woods exploring for hours and didn't get in trouble as long as we got back in time for dinner.

I rode my bike or walked to school. There weren't any moms lined up in their cars around the block dropping off their kids. In Jersey if you lived more than 2 miles from school you could take the school bus, otherwise you were on your own.
We also participated heavily in sports like baseball and touch football. I could catch really well but was a so-so hitter. Later I also got into basketball and loved playing pickup games. But I never made any organized teams because I was a skinny little runt. I reached 6'0" after a growth spurt at the end of my sophomore year in high school, and weighed about 145. Through a heroic effort over that summer I lifted weights and drank protein-rich shakes and managed to bulk up to 160, or just skinny instead of string bean.

I was also heavily into bicycling as a kid, mostly for getting around. My first bike was a little one with 20" wheels- just a small version of the typical heavy single speed "paperboy" bikes back then. This was way before bmx bikes, and even before the Schwinn Stingray had been introduced. I graduated to a larger 24" bike, but when I outgrew that I got my first "English racer". Now that was exciting. Raleigh exported a bunch of touring bikes with the famous Sturmey-Archer 3 speed hub gears, but we thought they were racers because they had gears and were lighter than the klunkers we were riding. Mine was a low-end knock off of the Raleighs, but I loved it and zoomed around everywhere on it. I couldn't imagine needing more gears- one for uphill, one for flat, and one for downhill, what more could you want? Like most kids, I abandoned biking at 15 or so when I started dreaming about cars instead.

With all the activity walking and biking everywhere, and all the sprinting that naturally occurs in the sports I played, you'd think I was in great shape. But I could not run very far continuously, so I guess you need to train for that, even as a kid. I remember my junior high had a special track and field day where anyone could enter various events. I figured I was too slow for the sprints so I thought I'd enter the quarter mile (which to me seemed like a long distance race). I went to the track after school and barely managed to run one lap, slowly, and decided entering the event was probably not a good idea.

I was not into running as an enjoyable activity on its own, just in support of organized sports. I did manage to work up to running about a mile and a half before trying out for basketball and football in high school, and thought that meant I was in fantastic shape. I lettered in football in high school, which is hard to believe in retrospect. I might have made a decent, if not particularly fast, wide receiver. But our team didn't have wide receivers, so I had to try to be a tight end, which didn't work out because skinny kids can't block too well. I ended up mostly holding the dummy bags and getting run over a lot by big people in practice. I never quit though, hung in there through senior year and got my football letter. Not sure if that showed mental toughness, poor judgement, or both.

With my build I would have been better suited trying to be a distance runner and going out for cross country or track. I remember being inspired by the exploits of Jim Ryun and his legendary duels with Kip Keino. But for some reason it never occurred to me to try it out.

Physical activity among adults was already pretty low by then. Few people went to gyms, and cars had largely displaced walking among adults in suburbia. There were exceptions- one car families were more common, so if the breadwinner took the car, the rest of the family had to take buses, walk, or ride bikes. So my Grandma would sometimes walk to the market wheeling a little shopping cart, or would send one of us kids on errands. All the grownups I knew were all pretty sedentary and some were overweight (though not bad by today's standards). The exception was my Uncle Din, who was way ahead of his time because he walked an hour a day. He was quite fit and trim, but I think the other adults thought all that walking was a bit odd.

One thing has definitely changed for the better since the days of my youth. It seemed like everybody smoked back then. My mom and all my aunts and uncles did (except Uncle Din). At family gatherings we'd be sitting around the table after eating and there would be a huge cloud of smoke. If one of the kids waved a hand in front of their face to try and breath fresh air we'd be told "stop showing off". There were cigarette ads everywhere, on TV, on billboards, in magazines. In restaurants they had no-smoking sections that were often not physically separated from the smoking section, so the air wasn't much better. We couldn't sit at them anyway since we always had at least one smoker (Mom) with us. I do not miss any of that. Years later my Mom ended up dying of a Bronchiectasis, a type of chronic obstructive pulmonary disease (COPD). She had quit smoking by her early fifties but by then it was too late. Anyone that smokes nowadays and thinks they're being cool or sophisticated, think again. It's just stupid.

I got accepted to the US Military Academy at West Point after high school and went for plebe (freshman) year. I was inspired to go there because I admired Uncle Din, who was a career army officer, and had an older cousin John who was a historian and would regale me with stories of the heroic military exploits of my ancestors. I had also been born at the military hospital at West Point: my father was serving in the navy in the Korean War so my Mom could go to military facilities for free, and the closest to where she lived was at West Point.

I showed up on July 1, 1970 for "beast barracks", which is what plebes endure the summer before the school year starts. I found it to be mentally challenging. Plebes are subjected to a lot of psychological abuse, the philosophy (at least back then) being to first break you down so they can then build you back up to be a leader. But I didn't find it overly demanding physically, I actually enjoyed doing "Army stuff". We'd go on long hikes with heavy packs carrying our M14 rifles, and camp out in a rural part of upstate New York, where we qualified in marksmanship and did other army maneuvers. Back at West Point we did a lot of light calisthenics, and lots of marching. We did parades every Saturday, and it was inspiring marching in precision to John Philips Souza music.

I played intramural sports like basketball and volleyball. What I did find physically challenging was gym class. This was not your typical college PhysEd. We did survival swimming, wrestling, gymnastics, and boxing.

I made it through plebe year, doing well academically and getting a great math education. You have to attend rigorous math courses six days a week, and end up fulfilling the math requirements for engineering in only one year. Unfortunately, this was not a good time to be a West Point. Morale in the army was low because of the unpopularity of the Vietnam War, and that had spread to the academy. It was a very cynical place, far from the gung ho attitude you'd expect, the outlook was to try to skate by. I'm sure it's not that way now, this was just a bad time to be there. That was what got to me, not the hazing, which isn't pleasant but you learn pretty quickly not to take personally. So I was pretty disillusioned and decided to quit even though I made it to the end of plebe year. I have a lot of respect for people who serve in the military and for West Point, but I was just there at the wrong time.

A good thing that came out of West Point is that when I was home on Christmas leave I met a beautiful young woman named Karen Orban. We corresponded when I went back, and she came up to visit a couple of times, and we fell in love. We were an item after I came back home and got married three years later when I finished undergraduate school. We've been married more than 44 years, so that worked out pretty well. After West Point I ended up going to Rutgers University (the state university of New Jersey) to become a civil engineer. I enjoyed it and did well in academics, especially my science and engineering courses. That summer before school started was the first time I got badly out of shape. I wasn't participating in any sports and hadn't found any new activities I liked, so I wasn't very active. Finally the lifetime skinny kid was able to start putting on weight, but more around the midsection than where I would have liked. I felt guilty about not exercising so tried running, but it felt like a chore and I couldn't get motivated.

Fortunately once school started I managed to remain pretty active physically, playing a lot of pickup basketball and intramural volleyball. I also had a cool old professor that had a vacation mobile home in the Catskills in upstate New York and would take Rutgers students up there to hike some of the "3500s" (peaks in the Catskills over 3500 feet). This was my first experience in the mountains and I loved it. The excess weight came off when I got active again.

Activity in adulthood

Upon graduation Karen and I moved to Camp Hill, Pa (across the Susquehanna River from Harrisburg) where I worked in civil engineering with a consulting firm. I had trouble fitting being active around a full time work schedule, so I again got out of shape. I tried to counter it by taking up running, partially inspired by Dr. Ken Cooper's <u>Aerobics</u> which had come out in 1968 and had an aerobic point system. I didn't enjoy running much because I went too fast. You could earn "points" more quickly by going faster, so I figured it was more efficient earning the points at a faster rate. It did not occur to me that it might be more enjoyable to go at a more comfortable pace.

I also got my first 10 speed bike, a cheap department store version with crappy brakes and shoddy shifting, but I still enjoyed taking it on rides on the bike paths along the Susquehanna and on some islands in the middle of it.

After a couple of years, we moved to the San Francisco bay area in Northern California, where I found a job in Palo Alto with another consulting firm. We lived in Mountain View, a little over 10 miles from work. Commuting by car or transit (only busses were available at the time) turned out to be pretty awful at rush hour, so my co-worker Malcolm, who happened to be a former bike racer from Scotland, suggested I take my bike. The commute took about 40 minutes one way, less time than it took by car or bus, and I got a nice workout and arrived relaxed to work in the morning and home at night. Malcolm also convinced me to ditch my cheap bike and get a good one, so for the first time in my life I bought a bike from an actual bike store. It was still at the lower end of the price range but it seemed quite luxurious to me. My daily commute added up to more than 100 miles a week of biking, so I thought I was in great shape.

My company formed an adult-ed basketball team, and I couldn't wait to impress everybody with how fit I was. I got my comeuppance at our first practice when I got gassed after the first few times up and down the floor. This taught me the concept that training is specific- bicycling doesn't get you fit for running, and 100 miles at a steady brisk pace does not get you ready for sprinting.

I stayed with the consulting firm for two years, then was fortunate enough to receive a fellowship to Stanford for my master's year, where I switched from civil to mechanical engineering. After the masters, I continued on to get a PhD, which was paid for by graduate research assistantships. Karen and I lived off campus 12 miles away so I continued with my bike commuting. On nice days I'd sometimes take the long way home through the foothills of the Santa Cruz Mountains.

After graduating I got a research position with the National Bureau of Standards (since renamed the National Institute of Science and Technology) in Boulder, Colorado. The research there was mostly on using fracture mechanics to determine scientific weld quality standards in pipelines and naval vessels, and was challenging and fun, and my coworkers were good colleagues and friends.

And Boulder itself was great, it's an outdoor enthusiast's and athlete's mecca. I continued my biking, going on long weekend rides (including a century, or 100 mile ride) with the biking group associated with the Colorado mountain club. My favorite ride was the mountain loop which had been used as part of the Coors classic bike race at that time. I did this with my boss at the Bureau, who was more than 10 years older than me but still fitter. It was 93 miles through the mountains, including a stop in the town of Nederland at a firemen's' pancake breakfast. Unfortunately we still had over a thousand feet of climbing to do, for which the pancakes provided fuel but also a dead weight in our stomachs. I think the racers did this route in about 3 ½ hours (minus the pancakes) but it took us a few hours longer. But it was harder to ride through the winters in Boulder, which include high winds, cold, and snow (Colorado mountain club called their winter rides the "frostbite series").

So I also got into hiking in the hills west of Boulder. I could walk for a quarter mile, from the townhouse we rented to a trail in the Boulder mountain park system, then about 45 minutes later I'd be at a vantage point where I could see peaks of the continental divide. Fitting that in in the morning before work is a great way to start your day. On longer hiking trips, friends and I did three of Colorado's 14'ers (fourteen thousand foot peaks). Long's peak was the most challenging. The first time we tried it was with a mixed group of fitness levels, and the pace wasn't fast enough, so we ran out of time: We were within view of the summit but got turned away by a thunderstorm that was striking the top with lightning. Thunderstorms are a common summer occurrence in the front range of the Rockies. On a second try, the guys I was with were all in good shape and we set a fast pace but it still took several hours. The altitude really got to me as we neared the peak. There's a last steep section called "home stretch", that's like climbing a few flights of stairs, which took forever. Step, step, gasp, gasp, repeat. It turned out to be a nice day at the top that day so we hung out there for a while, and I ended up with a bad altitude headache.

My favorite 14'er was Mt. Missouri. I remember it had a long narrow ridge you had to scamper along near the summit with spectacular views- just don't look down if you aren't fond of heights. And on the way down one of my buddies, an experienced rock climber, taught us how to glissade down a scree slope. You take giant steps and intentionally slide before the next step. Fast and fun! I didn't have as much trouble with altitude on that hike because we'd been backpacking a couple of days at over 10,000 feet so I was better acclimatized

I also hiked rim-to-rim in the Grand Canyon with my brother Bill and his friends. That took all day, and the logistics were also tricky. A friend of my brother's was going fishing north of the Canyon, so he offered us a ride. We drove up from Phoenix, dropped a car off at the south rim, then he drove us all the way around to the north rim, through the night, while we tried to sleep in the back. Starting on the North rim in the morning, we hiked across, and came up the South Kaibab trail, which, by the time we got to it, was in the dark. Not a good idea, as this trail is used to take tourists up from Phantom Ranch at the bottom on mules, and mule urine smells pretty nasty. Bill's friend was in the lead because he had the only flashlight. So we'd hear him call out warnings. "Mule piss, left!"… "Mule Piss, right!" Then he'd miss one and we'd hear a splash followed by "Oh, x!@x&!".

I also took up running in Boulder, for the first time grasping the concept that if you take it easy it can be fun. It was especially nice along the Mesa trail in the large mountain park above Boulder. I did my first 10K race, the Bolder Boulder, which had some good bands along the course and was fun at the easy pace I ran it.
I then took a job with IBM research in south San Jose, back in the San Francisco bay area. We moved to a place in a rural area south of the research facility, in the hills west of Morgan Hill. It wasn't practical for me to commute by bike on a regular basis, because although the local roads in the area are great for riding, they have narrow shoulders, and I wasn't comfortable next to the insanely fast traffic at rush hour.

So I gave up biking for running, and got more heavily into it this time. Over about the next 20 years I ran countless 10K's, and three marathons (in 1987, 1993, and 2000). As you can see each time it took several years for me to forget how much the last one hurt, and convince myself that doing another would be fun.

The first marathon was San Francisco 1987. I did pretty well, clipping off comfortable 9:00 minute miles for 3 hours, then after mile 20 I fell apart- my quads were shot. I remember it felt like somebody was sticking an ice pick in my thigh with each step. It felt a lot better if I walked, so I did so for much of the last 6 miles, finishing in 4 hours 37 minutes.

I also did some hiking while at IBM. One of my favorites was to the top of half dome in Yosemite, which I did with a friend in a long day. I also enjoyed doing Mt. Tallac, the tallest mountain in the Lake Tahoe basin. Half-dome is 8839 feet, Mt Tallac 9738. I had no altitude problems on either of these, so I guess there's a big difference between 10000 and 14000 feet.

After a few years at IBM I left to establish, along with 3 coworkers, a small Silicon Valley start-up that developed analysis software for mechanical engineers. Unfortunately this involved trading a short car commute on rural roads for a long and nasty commute to north San Jose. I kept up my running, and for the most part my sanity, by running at lunch hour and doing longer runs on my days off. I did sign up for the Napa marathon in 1992 and made sure I did some longer training runs. This time I made it to mile 22 before the quads gave out again, so I had to walk about 4 miles, finishing in 4:09, which turned out to be my lifetime PR. A couple of months later, with all the training I'd put in for the marathon, I was able to run a PR of 43:21 in a 10K, which also ended up being a lifetime PR. I was 40 that year, so I guess I really was over the hill, at least speedwise, after that. It's funny that I remember those numbers so precisely all these years later, there must be something about running organized events that makes you retain the times.

After about seven years our little company was acquired by a larger company, PTC. After a couple of years with them, I decided I was burned out from the start-up experience, and left to try freelancing on my own and some teaching of engineering. This gave me a looser schedule which allowed me to pursue outdoor hobbies like running and hiking, and some kayaking in the summer.

I took some lessons and qualified to rent sea-touring kayaks, which are faster than the ones they rent to novices, and can handle rougher weather. I also took a surf-zone course which was fun, we had to learn to launch through larger waves and land through larger surf. It's a good thing they make you wear a helmet for that, because on my first try landing, the surf picked me and my kayak up, turned it sideways, and dumped me on the beach, whacking my head in the sand. My favorite place to kayak was the length of Elkhorn Slough, about 10 miles round trip, with amazing wildlife including sea otters, sea lions, harbor seals, and many varieties of birds.

I gave the marathon one last shot, signing up for Portland, 2000. This time I was able to run the whole thing, even though the last few miles were uncomfortable. When your quads hurt, downhill running is actually more painful. I think it was around mile 23 that we crossed a bridge over the Willammette. After that a well-meaning bystander was cheering us on with "it's all downhill from here", not knowing that was not good news for me at the time. I slowly shuffled in with a 4:32.

After Portland I began to develop some pain in my right hip so I decided, somewhat belatedly, to do nothing longer than a half marathon. There were a lot of trail half marathons in the bay area at that time so I tried a couple of those. They were much more enjoyable than marathons, still enough of a challenge but not enough to fall apart at the end. And they were in great locations like up in the Santa Cruz Mountains. In retrospect I wish I had done more of those instead and stopped after the first marathon. For me at least, one marathon is a great thing to check off your bucket list. More than one meant I was a slow learner.

Fighting off Decrepitude

The hip pain continued, and at the age of 48 I was diagnosed with osteoarthritis in my right hip. It became a priority at this point to minimize further damage to the thin layer of remaining cartilage, hopefully to avoid needing a hip replacement. My orthopedic doctor was a running enthusiast herself, and said I could continue running but only gentle short runs. I think she had a moral dilemma here, as I really shouldn't be doing activities that cause impact to the damaged cartilage anymore, but she couldn't bring herself to condemn me to a life without running. But she also recommended coming up with alternatives that were lower impact. I read all I could about arthritis and exercise, and spent several months trying out different things. For a while I had a cardio routine on indoor machines at the gym but it was not too enjoyable after being used to outdoor exercise in beautiful surroundings. I remember an older friend at the gym teasing me that now I had to be inside with the old farts. I laughed, but I found this very depressing. So for a few weeks I gutted out working out at the gym, and found out what it's like for everyone that doesn't have a physical activity they enjoy.

I did find walking outdoors to be pleasant. You can make walking into a better workout by adding the upper body to it by using poles or hand weights (described in chapter 3). But at the time I couldn't go very briskly with my bum hip. I tried roller blading but it still made my hip sore. I also did a few too many faceplants, perhaps a lesson would have helped.

I also tried roller skiing. It felt great when I was doing it, I imagined I was a cross country racer! But because I developed some back pain, I asked my wife to take a video of me doing it so I could check out my posture. Posture was ok, but the video showed how ridiculously slow I was moving. That was a bit discouraging, plus I was clumsy enough to fall on a couple of occasions.

Finally I decided to retry biking. I figured it would be ok on the country roads near my house as long as I avoided rush hour. I started out with a cheap department store "comfort" bike to make sure it was really going to stick, then after a few months I gave that away and treated myself to a nice hybrid from Gary Fisher (when he still had his own company, which was later acquired by Trek). I had a bit of a problem with comfort (butt and neck issues), so I later tried recumbent biking. After experimenting with a couple of models, I finally found the "Rans Rocket" short wheelbase recumbent to be comfortable on long rides. I even got a front fairing to make it go faster. I'm sure it was a bit of a weird sight out on our country roads. I also rode with a group on longer rides, who were tolerant of my odd bike, though I did get teased a bit. So I got satisfaction on windy flat sections, when they would tuck in behind me to take advantage of the draft from my fairing. Later I switched to a more aerodynamic recumbent, the Strada, from Bacchetta, which didn't need a fairing to go fast, so I didn't look quite as weird.

With all the various contraptions that I tried, a neighbor asked me if I was a product tester. I think it made her nervous when I said no, because that was probably the only explanation she had come up where I might be reasonably sane.

Once I got seriously into biking I decided I needed a challenge so started looking for a century ride to sign up for. That's kind of the bicyclist's equivalent of a marathon. Then I discovered Clarence Bass's website (www.cbass.com). Clarence is a both a former Olympic weightlifter and bodybuilder with great advice on training. At the time he was in his early 60s and still in amazing health and condition; he still is now, at 80!

He recommends finding a challenge to motivate your training. But I noticed his personal challenges are quite a bit shorter, like trying to set a good time for his age group rowing 500 meters on the Concept2 rowing machine. People from around the world have been posting their times for years, long before there was anything like Strava for other sports. Rowing 500 is an event that takes less than 2 minutes but leaves you totally gassed if you give it your all. Making marginal improvements in your time is a lot of work. Clarence's site also introduced me to high intensity interval training, a challenging but enjoyable way to get faster. I like to do 8x30 sec sprints standing on my bike, with about 60 sec recovery in between. Great workout. I don't need to run marathons anymore for mental toughness. When you get to the 5th sprint or so, it builds enough toughness fighting to keep going. The short challenge I came up with is timing myself climbing a local hill on my bike, which is a tough 60 seconds or so.

One positive thing that happened during my depressing exercise-as-a-chore period (before I got back into biking) was that I learned to enjoy strength training more. I found the best way for me to get inspired to do it was to think about outdoor activities that need upper body strength, like cross-country skiing and kayaking, in which I participated seasonally.

In 2008 Karen and I found a nice house close to downtown Morgan Hill. It took a couple of years to sell our country place, and in the interim we had two mortgages and things were a bit tight financially. So I returned to PTC and worked there until they closed their San Jose office in 2013, after which I returned to freelancing. Biking near our little downtown is a lot better, there are many bike lanes and quiet roads, and I am near to the Coyote creek path on which you can bike car-free for many miles (47 miles round trip if I go the whole length).

I set up a garage gym for strength training, with dumbbells and also resistance bands. I would just add more bands as I got stronger, which eventually required getting more heavy duty handles when I broke the plastic ones I started with. A nice tangible sign of progress when you start breaking stuff while strength training! I also added a short yoga routine at night that I had cobbled together from classes and books I had read over the years. This is great for stress relief, but also keeps me limber. There is some controversy over the kind of static stretching done in yoga, as in whether it is a good warmup or the best way to increase your flexibility. But I don't use it for either of those reasons, it's for relaxation and to prevent getting stiffer with age. I'm a lot slower than I was a few decades ago, but thanks to my evening yoga routine I am not any stiffer.

Around 2010, I supplemented all of the above by joining an outrigger canoe club In San Jose. I had been kayaking in Monterey bay and noticed their local club out practicing and it looked like fun, so I looked into it and found there was a San Jose club about 15 miles north of my home. We practiced on some weeknights and Saturday mornings, and in the summers attended regattas in various parts of Northern California, where we raced against other clubs in 6-person canoes. This was very vigorous exercise, but fun because of the camaraderie. I found you can push yourself a lot harder when you don't want to let your crewmates down. We did races that involved 180 degree turns, a tricky task in 44 foot long canoes. After the turn we'd have lost all momentum and the steersman (or woman) would yell out "dead water, get us moving!" Even though your arms would be burning and feel ready to fall off at that point, you could still dig deeper and respond.

All in all I appeared to be aging gracefully and staying in decent shape, but friends kept nagging me that I was starting to limp. I also was having back pain. I kept insisting the problem was not my hip, because part of my yoga routine was a hip stretch, which I could do just fine. What I didn't realize was that my hip was actually almost locked, and when I thought I was stretching it I was actually torqueing my back. It had been about 10 years since my arthritis diagnosis and unbeknownst to me, the hip had continued to degenerate.

I finally went to an excellent sports medicine doc, Dr. Jeffrey Blue. As soon as I walked into his office for what I thought would be my back examination he said "how long has your hip been that bad"? After an x-ray proved the back was just fine, he focused on my hip. He tried sending me to PT but the joint was too far gone so he referred me to an amazing surgeon, Dr. Nicholas Abidi, who is one of the minority of surgeons that does hip replacements using the anterior approach (accessing the joint through the front instead of the back) which minimizes muscle damage and has much shorter rehab time.

My first visit with Dr. Abidi was entertaining as well as educating. Having quickly looked at the bilateral x-ray of my hips, he came in and started manipulating my left hip and said "this is really bad, we need to fix this". I replied "Uh, Doc, it's the other one". So he went and looked at the x-ray again and said "wow the right one is even worse". Then he was happy to find out I was an engineer, so he could explain to me, in technical terms, the advantages of the anterior approach to surgery. But when I asked him how long I could wait before surgery he put technicalities aside, looked me in the eye and said "you have to do this now or you're going to have a shitty outcome". It turns out my hip was so far gone that the ball and socket were starting to fuse together. When you try to take out a fused joint prior to replacing it, damage can occur to the socket leading to "a shitty outcome".

He had an opening in 8 days so we scheduled it. Dr. Abidi operates at Dominican Hospital in Santa Cruz, about 20 miles from our house as the crow flies but 46 miles as the car drives because it's on the other side of the Santa Cruz mountains. So we booked a hotel there, for Karen and me to stay the first night, and for Karen to stay the rest of my time in the hospital. In May 2012, I had the surgery, which went without a hitch.

It consisted of removing the portion of the thigh bone (femur) that bends over toward the "ball" of the hip joint (technically the "femoral neck and head"), and placing a metal (cobalt chrome) implant inside the socket in the pelvis (known as the "actetabulum"). The correct size titanium implant is then chosen, which is inserted down into the femur. Over time the bone will grow around it and grab on tightly to it so it is well-secured. This implant replaces the part of the femur that was removed, including the ball of the joint. In between the two metal pieces a layer of low friction and highly wear-resistant plastic is placed. This wear layer should be good for about 25 years if you minimize impact to the joint. If necessary it can be replaced in a revision operation, but it is best to treat the hip right to postpone that as long as possible, so running is still not a good idea.

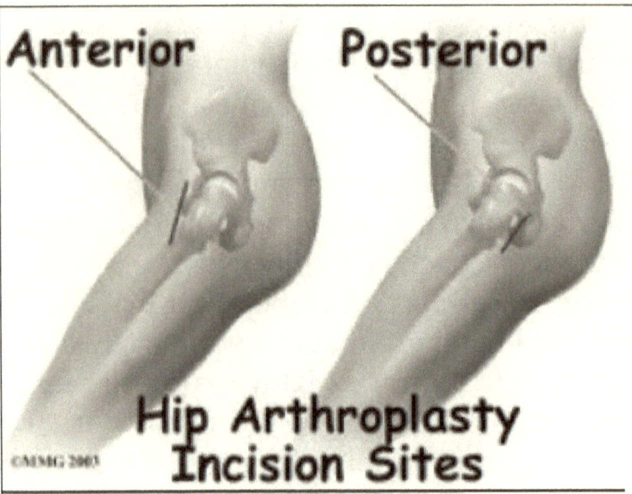

In the anterior approach, the surgeon comes in through the front of the leg, sneaking in between two of the quadriceps muscles.

"Arthroplasty" is the medical term for joint replacement.

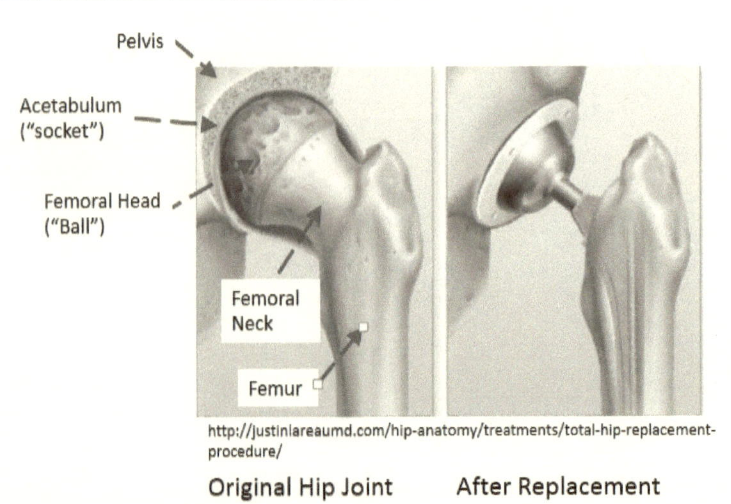

The Surgeon removes the femoral neck and head. The metal insert is shoved down the femur. The surgeon cleans the surface of the acetabulum and inserts a metal cup. There is a low-friction wear resistant plastic lining between the new ball on the insert and the new cup. In my case the cup was cobalt-chrome, the insert titanium, and the lining ultra-high molecular weight polyethylene.

This was my first experience with major surgery (actually with any surgery at all except removing wisdom teeth). It was a great experience, being taken care of by highly competent people. The morning of the surgery, 5 AM sharp, we did some check-in paperwork. Then I went through pre-op, cleaning and prepping of the surgical site, and talking to the anesthesiologist. It was cold in the hospital, since it's close to the coast, and I started shivering when I got on the gurney to wait to get wheeled in.

But then the nurse put a warmed-up blanket on me. "Ah, is this a hospital or a spa"? They started an IV drip as I was getting wheeled in, and I zonked out right after we went through the double doors leading to surgery.

I remember waking up in recovery and thinking "wow, I'm lying flat on my back and it doesn't hurt". For several years, the bum hip joint had tugged at my back so it hurt to lay flat unless I propped up my knees. This was the first sign things were about to get a lot better.It's astonishing how quickly they want you up and moving after surgery these days. No more "bed rest". My physical therapist got me out of bed, walking around the room, then sitting up in a chair, the afternoon of the surgery.

Unfortunately I fainted in the chair because I was still low on fluids after the surgery. My PT had been called away by a code blue, but I was lucky my friend Annie who has been to nursing school happened to be visiting. She saw my eyes roll up right before I conked out, and immediately jammed my shoulders to the back of the chair or I might have fallen. Karen ran out in the hallway and yelled for help and the cavalry came and got me back in bed.

This incident made me end up staying in the hospital 2 nights instead of just one. But they quickly solved the fluid problem with IV, and I was soon walking up and down the halls, and had to also practice on stairs since my house is two stories. For about 3 weeks until the hip is more recovered, you do stairs one leg at a time, leading with the "good leg" and following with the "bad" on the way up, and reversing that on the way down.

Not everything was great. There were the "itchies" that kept me awake at night, which were helped a bit by a Benadryl IV. And getting your catheter removed does not make my top ten list of fun things. But I received great care from competent and compassionate people. I made sure to always express my gratitude to all of them.

After 2 nights we went home, and it was great to be sleeping in my own bed. But sleeping turned out to be an issue for about a week. My body just felt "antsy" for a while, maybe it is a systemic reaction to major surgery, or maybe the drugs weren't totally out of my system. It's not like normal insomnia where your brain just won't shut up. I was happy, my mind was calm, I just couldn't sleep because my body felt weird.

Fortunately this went away fairly quickly. I started out at home with a walker that I only needed for a few days, after which I graduated to a cane for a few weeks. Even after the first few days, I noticed how great walking felt. No more back pain, and it felt like I was gliding on air without having a stiff hip in the way. To this day walking still feels great to me.

I did my PT exercises faithfully. You lose some strength in your glutes and abductors during the long period when your hip movement is impaired due to severe arthritis, and diligent work is required to get the strength back with exercises like "the clamshell". These may not be fun but are important. My doc told me lots of his patients don't bother with this and never get a proper gait back! I don't understand why you'd go to all this trouble to get the hip fixed then not do your homework to make sure you can walk right.

Though I was walking just fine, the hip is vulnerable in this period because the femur has not yet grabbed on tightly to the implant. So falling is not a good idea. For this reason I also had to avoid biking for about a month, although I was able to stationary cycle.

There was very little pain in this whole period. I think they may have given me some morphine the day of surgery but there was not much need for painkillers after that. After about a month I felt 100%. This was in contrast to friends I knew that had the traditional posterior hip surgery, which involves cutting through the glute muscles, who had a lot more discomfort and took up to a year to rehab. There are also fewer movement limitations with the anterior surgery, like not being able to sit in a low chair or cross your legs because the new hip might dislocate.

This led to a funny incident when a P.T. came to check out my house and was saying things like "That chair's too low, and you need a toilet booster seat. Oh, never mind, I forgot you had the anterior surgery". I found out from the pathology report of my removed hip that I had a condition called "avascular necrosis": there is insufficient blood supply to the "ball" of the hip joint, which causes the cartilage to prematurely degenerate, leading to arthritis.

This meant the left hip was not far behind the right, as Dr. Abidi had already noticed on my x-ray. I probably could have waited as much as a year or so, but decided to go ahead and do the left as soon as it was a good idea, which turned out to be four months after the first operation. This one went even smoother since Karen and I were now experienced at it. No "itchies" this time, as Dr. Abidi expected that was due to my anesthesia the first time, so he made sure the anesthesiologist tweaked my meds. I was discharged after only one night because I didn't have the fainting issue this time. I had a similar experience with rehab, again 100% recovered after a month.

The second hip was done in September 2012 when I was 59. The following January I would turn 60 so I treated myself to a really nice present to celebrate my rehab and 60th birthday at the same time: A Bike Friday super-pro. This is a travel bike that fits in a suitcase but is also a high quality roadbike. I've ridden in senior game time trials with it and it also has really low gears so can climb like a mountain goat (although it would help if it had a more powerful engine). My biggest climb on it so far has been the Mt. Diablo challenge (3249 ft.). I love that little bike, with its small wheels and snappy acceleration. Kids love it too, I get a lot of "hey mister, cool bike!"

After rehabbing the 2nd hip, I got extra-enthused about my
training and managed to tear my Achilles tendon. Fortunately
a partial tear can heal itself without surgery if you immobilize
it, so now I was stuck in a boot for a few months and had to
do more P.T. I stubbornly kept riding my bike. I thought I
looked like an idiot but I got compliments for my tenacity. My
wife was very supportive of my riding- I'd tell her "I'm
committed to biking", and she'd say "Yes, you should be
committed".

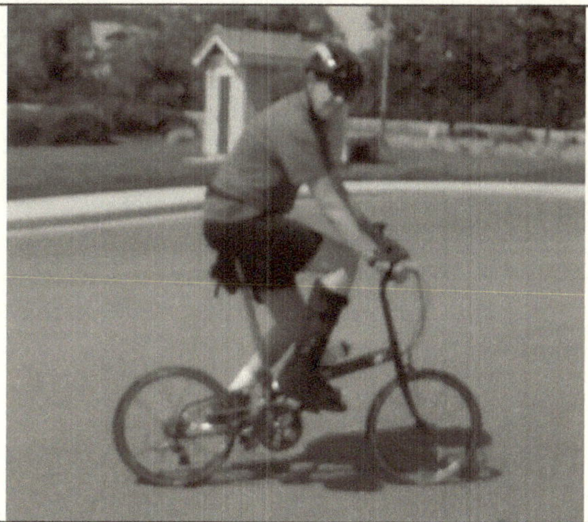

Too stubborn to quit- riding while in boot with torn Achilles tendon

I stopped going to the canoe club during my hip adventures.
Kayaking and recreational canoeing (or stand-up paddling)
are fine but outrigger canoe racing was getting hard on my
back so I never did return to it. But I still had plenty to keep
me active. I discovered that standing up to pedal on a bike
feels similar to running and is comfortable, so I sold my
recumbent and just did conventional biking with a lot of
standing up. I also could now walk briskly without hip issues,
including doing it with hand weights or poles to get a better
workout. I also got into doing time trial races, informal local
ones as well as the "Bay Area senior games".

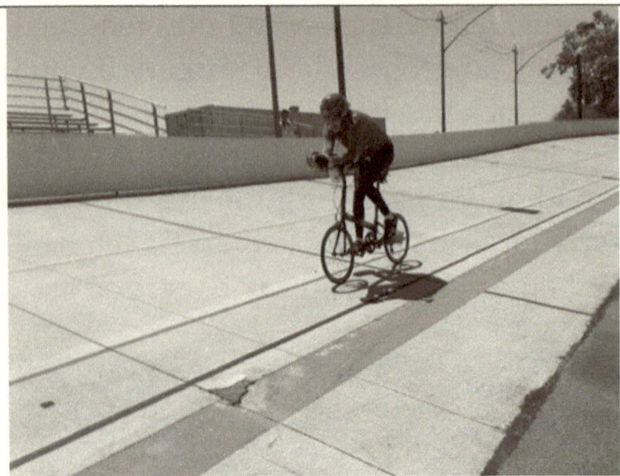
Me on Superpro at Hellyer Velodrome in San Jose (seconds before crashing- oops!)

We have a concrete velodrome in Hellyer Park in San Jose, the only one in Northern California, built in 1963 for the Pan Am games and used for the 1972 trials for the US Olympic Team. Once a year users are allowed to ride regular bikes instead of track bikes on it.

They let you just try it out but also have short time trials where you get up to speed on one lap, then are timed for the second lap, where you go as hard as you can. I had a great time doing this until I crossed the finish line, and tried to come up out of the aerobars on my bike into the normal handlebar position. While still at high speed and one hand off the bars, the front wheel hit a bump in the track which sent it wobbling wildly and I went down spectacularly.

This was my first experience with severe road rash, which I got when I scraped my right hip and butt during the fall. If you watch events like the Tour de France, you've seen amazing crashes, then the victims covered in gauze the next day, ready to race again. Now I found out what they really go through. I was too sore and stiff for a couple of days to even think about getting back on a bike or even do brisk walking, then it got a little better and I could move around a bit more. But the worst part was the itching! I was unable to sleep for several nights, because every time I'd start to nod off it felt like somebody was sticking me with pins. The itching receded a little after several days, so I could sleep, but the wound didn't heal completely for about 10 weeks. I don't care if you're in good shape, skin takes a lot longer to heal when you're 62. Karen made me promise no more velodromes. She's a really nice nurse when I'm rehabbing, as long as I'm obedient.

Heart Surgery and Rehab

After my road rash escapade I got back into working out full blast and felt things were going well. The first intimation something was wrong was when I did the senior games time trial again, and my performance was a lot worse than the previous year. I seemed to get badly out of breath after several minutes at high intensity. Over the next couple of months, this happened more than once, usually when hiking or biking up steep hills, which I knew in the past I'd been able to handle just fine.

I went to Dr. Blue for a checkup and he thought he heard a heart murmur, so he referred me to a cardiologist. Bingo! An echocardiogram (ultrasound of the heart) revealed "moderate aortic stenosis". This means the aortic valve, which is the one leading out of the heart into the aorta, to supply blood to the entire body, was not opening enough.

Heart valves are what engineers (and plumbers) call "check valves": they passively open under pressure to let the blood flow out, then slam shut to prevent backflow. Many times per minute, tens of thousands of times per day. The heart has an ingenious mechanism for doing this: there are 3 leaflets of tissue in a circle. They open leaving a wide area for blood flow, then slam shut to prevent backflow ("regurgitation" in medicalese).

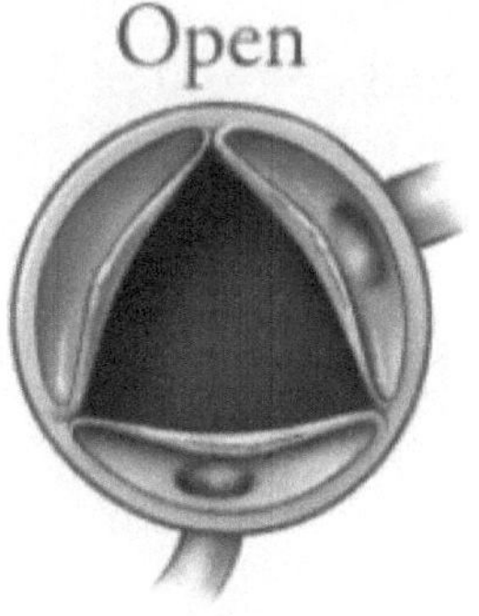 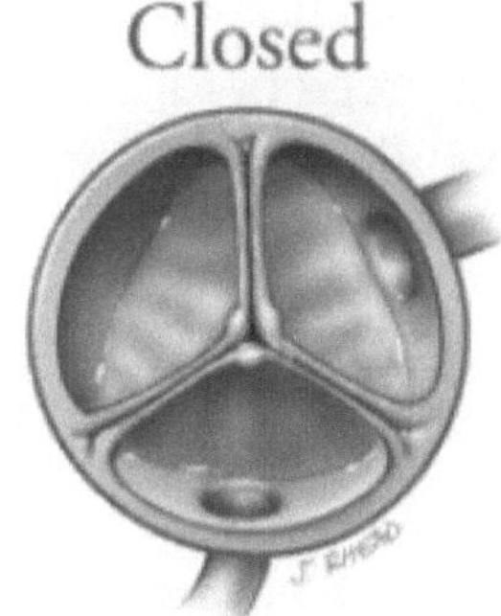

Healthy aortic valve (www.intermountainhealthcare.org)

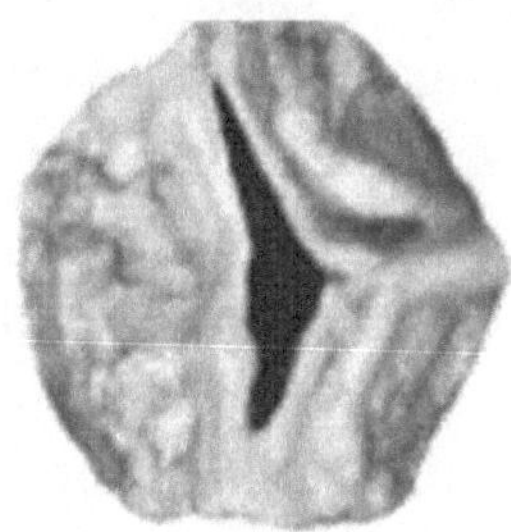

Bicuspid aortic valve with calcification. Contrast this fully open position with that of the healthy valve (www.heartsurgeryinfo.com)

Three things can go wrong. As we age, calcium deposits form on the leaflets and they get stiffer, so the valve doesn't open as much as it should. The second is a congenital condition where the valve has only two leaflets, known as a bicuspid valve. This does not open properly your entire life, but maybe opens enough so you get by. Then as you get older and it calcifies it goes bad more quickly than a normal valve. The first two issues cause stenosis, where the valve doesn't open enough. The third problem is when the valve does not close properly and leaks, causing backflow, for which the medical term is regurgitation. I had stenosis but not regurgitation. My echo test could not visualize the valve well enough to tell if it was bicuspid but my cardiologist suspected it was, because I had significant stenosis already at the relatively young age of 63.

A normal aortic valve opens to about 2.5 to 4 cm^2, while with moderate stenosis it is about 1 to 1.5 cm^2, and it is considered severe when it goes below 1. Here's what that amount of opening looks like:

Mine was already like the middle picture, where the blood flow to my entire body had to squeeze through one of the fat straws for a Starbucks frappuccino instead of a garden hose. Later it would progress to the right picture, as small as a regular drinking straw. The first follow-up test was a treadmill stress test where they take your ekg while ramping up the speed and incline of the treadmill every couple of minutes. I ended up running briskly up a steep grade with my heart rate at 171, so I thought I had passed with flying colors. But my cardiologist noticed some arrhythmias at higher heart rate and said I could still exercise but keep it under 145. I started to monitor that with an old-school heart monitor with a chest strap.

Next he sent me for a "calcium score" which gives an idea of how much calcium is in your coronary arteries. I flunked that test, which concerned him even more than the heart valve, because it meant I might have coronary artery disease.

The next test was a stress-echocardiogram, an interesting experience: working out hard on the treadmill again, then the tech says "ok we're going to stop quickly" and immediately hits the stop button. I thought I was gonna fly through the front of the machine. She and the guy doing the echo then quickly got me laying down on my side while my chest was still heaving and he did a quick echo scan. The idea is to image the heart while it is working very hard. If any coronary arteries are even partially obstructed, the heart will have an abnormal shape, but mine turned out fine. This got me off the hook about the flunked calcium test.

So now I just had to follow up with regular echocardiograms every six months, which I ended up doing a couple of more times. During this period I kept exercising with the 145 limitation on heart rate, which still let me work out pretty hard, just no extended hard efforts. Short sprints and intervals were ok. I did get a repeat of the badly out of breath symptom, which I mentioned to my cardiologist, so I had to wear an "ecat" monitor ("external cardiac ambulatory telemetry") for a couple of weeks. This continuously checked my heart rhythm day and night. When it detected an arrhythmia, it sounded an alarm and I had it upload its signal to a monitoring site. This was actually by the antiquated procedure of dialing a number and letting the gizmo whistle its tone into the phone like I was sending a fax. It seems there are still a lot of areas in medicine where high tech has not quite caught up!

I managed to set the alarm off a couple of times while exercising hard. I guess the 145 limit was no longer strict enough. My cardiologist said the ecat had detected atrial fibrillation (afib) that comes on with exercise, probably a side effect of the bum heart valve. This is significant, because afib increases your risk of stroke. So now I was no longer allowed to do vigorous exercise, only brisk walking or equivalent.

In addition, my next echocardiogram showed I'd progressed to severe stenosis. It was now time for an angiogram. This is a somewhat invasive procedure, so it is not done for assessing heart valve disease until they're pretty sure it has progressed to severe.

They have to go in through an artery to insert a catheter for the procedure. They used to have to use the femoral artery in the groin, but if your arteries are in good enough shape they can now go in through the wrist. Fortunately that worked in my case. The angiogram showed my coronary arteries were clear, so the calcium score test had been a false alarm, which is actually quite rare.

Unblocked coronaries was the good news, the bad news was severe stenosis was confirmed, and it was time to get the valve replaced. I wanted the cardiac surgeon equivalent of Dr. Abidi so I did a lot of checking around. The best surgeon in my area turned out to be Dr. Vincent Gaudiani, who operates at El Camino hospital in Mountain View, Ca, a little over 30 miles from our house.

Valve replacement usually requires a "median sternotomy" which requires cutting your sternum completely in half. I had read about this possibly leading to long and uncomfortable rehab, so would have preferred a less invasive procedure. Dr. Gaudiani indeed does a procedure that only involves cutting the top portion of the sternum ("mini-sternotomy") and has shorter rehab. But because I also had afib, he needed to do the "Cox-Maze III" procedure while he had me open, and this requires the full sternum cut. He assured me this was the gold standard for treating afib that accompanies aortic stenosis. Dr. Gaudiani is a great guy and our consultation with him convinced Karen and me that I would be in good hands.

We did have one other choice to make- mechanical valve vs. biological tissue valve. The mechanical valve lasts forever but you need to be on blood thinners for life. And it makes a click that can be loud enough to bother some people. That would be a bummer, "uh, doc, that click is driving me nuts. Why don't you saw me back open and put the other valve in instead?" The tissue valves don't require blood thinners after you leave the hospital but can calcify after about 15-20 years (or fewer if you're unlucky) and need to be replaced.
But Dr. Gaudiani said this can be done by a minimally-invasive procedure, where a new valve is inserted via the femoral artery and deployed right inside the previous one (trans catheter aortic valve replacement, or TAVR). Or who knows what even better technique they'll have come up with in around 15 years. So we opted for tissue, which he said would either be porcine (pig) or bovine (cow) depending on the size valve I needed. Dr. Gaudiani made it clear we had to do this asap. Once it starts progressing, stenosis gets worse quickly. I'd probably be out of breath just walking around slowly within a few months, and could be dead in a year.

Ok, no dilly-dallying. We scheduled the surgery for August 11, 2017. A bonus was that we have dear friends that live a few blocks from the hospital. It happened they would be away the time of the surgery so they let Karen stay at their house.

Aside: (TMI Alert!): Aortic valve replacement and Cox-Maze III procedure

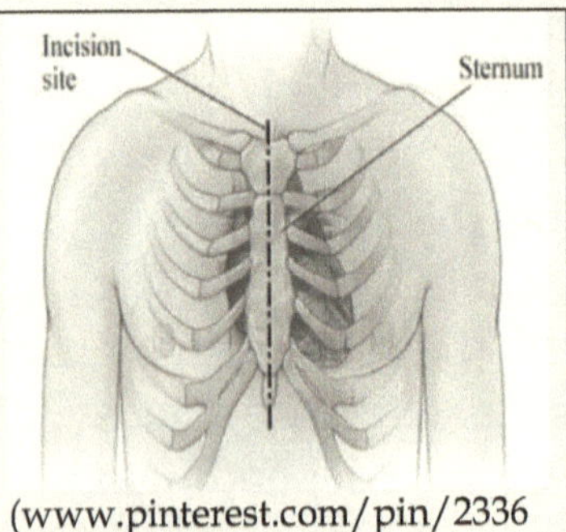

(www.pinterest.com/pin/2336
24491793903439)

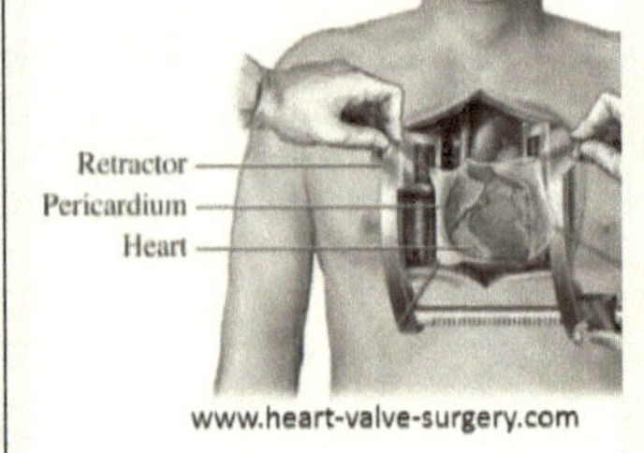

To have enough access to perform the Cox-Maze III procedure the surgeon has to cut the full length of the sternum ("median sternotomy"). Retractors pull the sternum out of the way during the procedure. The pericardium (the membrane enclosing the heart) is cut open to get to the heart. The surgeon cuts through the aorta to allow access to the valve. The old valve is removed, and a new one inserted (in my case a bovine tissue valve):

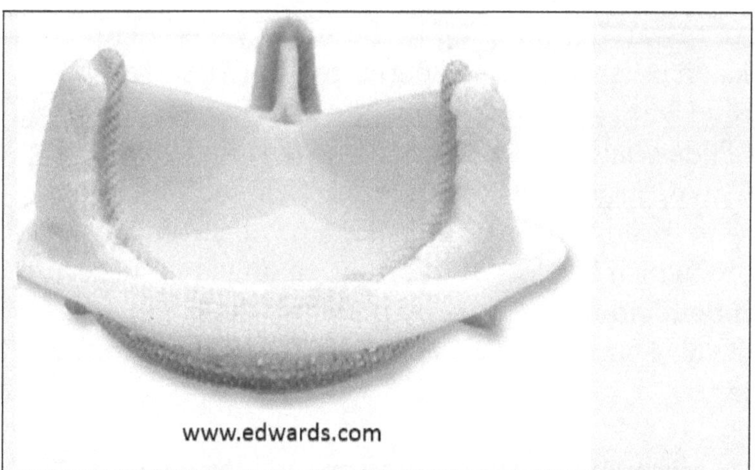

The new valve is sutured in place (there are also sutureless variations). The Cox-Maze III procedure is then performed if needed: The heart is pulled forward out of the pericardium. Talk about having your life in somebodies hands! Small nicks are made on the surface in strategic places and then sewn shut. This will leave scar tissue that disrupts the propagation of abnormal electrical signals that can cause Afib. This procedure evolved from the original procedure pioneered by Dr. James Cox.[190]

I did a lot of research leading up to the surgery, and read some books on other people's experiences. The first was <u>Opening My Heart: A Journey from Nurse to Patient and Back Again</u>, by Tilda Shalof[140]. The second was <u>The Patient's Guide To Heart Valve Surgery</u>, by Adam Pick[122]. This second book also led me to Adam's helpful website, www.heart-valve-surgery.com, which has lots of information on valve surgery, a surgeon finder, and many posts by patients who have undergone valve surgery. It was on Adam's site that I found Dr. Gaudiani.

This kind of research is very useful to get an idea what to expect. The downside is you have to be careful not to get freaked out by reading about some of the other people's experiences. Everyone is different, and "your results may vary". For example, both Tilda and Adam talked about a lot of post-operative pain in the sternum, and the need for narcotic pain meds. Adam had to be on them long enough to be concerned with getting addicted, but was able to wean himself off in time. Because of this I showed up for surgery having read books on pain management and with self-hypnosis tapes for pain relief, which turned out not to be needed. But overall it was good for me to have a solid idea what to expect, and I went into surgery with a positive attitude.

Here is my number one tip: put yourself in a good surgeon's hands and trust that it will go well. Do not focus on anything negative like the slight possibility of things going wrong in the surgery. Instead, focus on how great the outcome will be, and how much better you'll feel in a couple of months after some rehab.

I also did my best to stay in as good shape as I could leading up the surgery, given my heart rate limitations. I did a lot of strength training, knowing I'd be losing strength during the period after surgery when my "sternal precautions" would limit my upper body training. From my research I found it really helps to be fit, your chances of a good outcome are higher and you'll bounce back quicker. I remember reading one surgeon commenting "the ones who can walk a mile a day will do fine. It's the inactive ones I worry about". But I set my fitness bar somewhat higher than that.

With good attitude in place, we showed up bright and early on August 11, 2017 at El Camino hospital for the surgery. Actually it wasn't bright, it was still dark that early. But admission and prep for surgery went smoothly, and Karen's beautiful smiling face was the last thing I saw before I was wheeled through the double doors. My doc got the complex procedure shown above done in just over 90 minutes. Karen had asked what the shortest time surgery could possibly take and was told two hours. So she went to the cafeteria to get some coffee, and when she got back she was bummed that she had already missed the surgeon. But she was pleased to hear I was out already, which was a good sign. I woke up an hour or so later, and again saw Karen's smiling face. I figured it was good she was smiling, I must be ok.

I still had the tracheal tube that was used for the breathing machine during surgery so I couldn't talk. They make sure everything is stable before taking it out. I could only communicate with Karen and my nurse via thumbs up, thumbs down, or writing. "How you doing Rich?" Thumbs up. "Are you in pain"? Thumbs down.

We did have one scare, I started bleeding internally. It seemed like 20 or so people were buzzing around me working on it (Karen said later it was more like 4). I thought, gee this must be serious. Oh well, they look like they're pretty good at what they do, I'm sure they'll figure it out. Drugs help a lot at a time like this- I was still half in LA-LA-land from the anesthesia. It was a lot harder on Karen, who had to stay out of the way and watch without benefit of drugs. She also overheard them discussing I might need to be wheeled back into surgery if they didn't stop it soon. But they resolved it pretty quickly by injecting a clotting factor.

A while later I started having quite a bit of discomfort in my upper back. I figured it was just because I'd been laying on my back for so long, and maybe the nurse could rearrange me and fix it. I tried writing a note to Karen to explain this. I thought, she's a wonderful wife, but I can't believe how dense she's being! Later she showed me the notes and they made no sense whatsoever. It turned out I could only communicate by carefully writing one letter at a time. Eventually I got through and my nurse did try to reposition me but it didn't help. Shortly thereafter the breathing tube came out, which felt a bit weird but not particularly unpleasant. This was another ordeal people had warned about in my reading that turned out to be almost nothing in my case. Now I could talk (sort of, more like croak). But I didn't bother mentioning I was still in discomfort, because I didn't think we could do anything about it.

My back got worse by bedtime and I thought it was going to keep me awake. So my nurse gave me a narcotic in my IV and I slept fine. Next morning I woke with no pain. My surgeon's assistant came by and he thought the back issue was probably from excess fluid around my lungs (pleural effusion), a common side effect from my surgery. I was receiving intravenous diuretic to get rid of it, so it probably had gone down a lot overnight. He also said my removed heart valve had indeed been bicuspid as well as calcified.

That was the last narcotic I needed. The sternum did not hurt AT ALL. The only pain reliever I needed in the hospital was Tylenol, and that was for mild headaches, maybe a side effect of drugs I'd received. Nurses kept checking with me "any pain? Are you sure?" but I was amazingly fine. The post-op care I got after this surgery was even more incredible than for my hips, because you have to be monitored closely. I was in ICU the first two nights (because of the internal bleeding scare above they kept me there two nights instead of the usual one).

I insisted Karen go to our friend's house for a good night's sleep because my nurse was taking care of me just fine. After that you go to a step-down ward but vital signs are still on telemetry. There was one exception to the no pain- my chest hurt if I coughed or sneezed. This violently expands the chest cavity, causing the ribs to jerk on the sternum. But it didn't feel like bone pain, more like the soreness from a bad chest cold. The old school way to alleviate this is to teach you to hug a pillow when you feel a cough or sneeze coming on. The hospital gave me a heart shaped pillow for this, which I got all my nurses to sign, and still have as a keepsake.

But for coughing and sneezing, there's now a much better solution- the Heart Hugger! Believe it or not I'm not a paid spokesman but I loved this little gadget, which they issued me the first morning after my surgery.

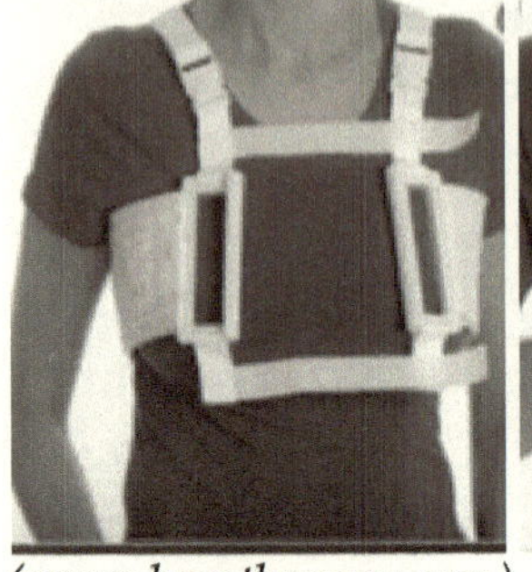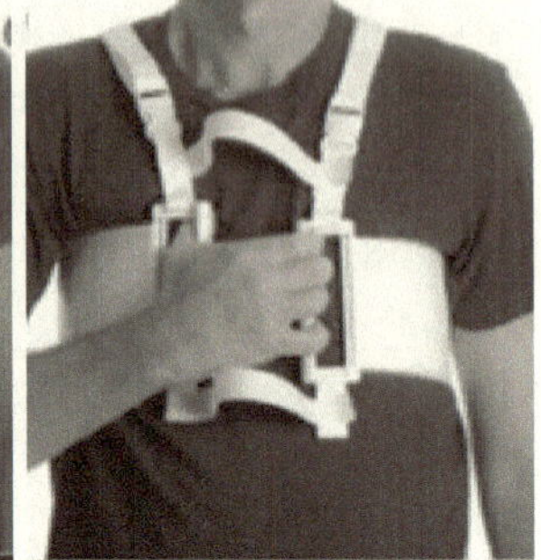

(www.hearthugger.com)

It's loose enough to let you breathe normally, but when a cough or sneeze comes on, you grab the straps and it supports you snugly, preventing pain. It was invented by a fellow engineer who himself had open heart surgery and thought there must be a better way than hugging a pillow. Clever, the design he came up with. If you are ever having this type of surgery I'd highly recommend checking with your surgeon to make sure they will be giving you this in the hospital. If not, you can buy it for yourself at the website- well worth it. What is pictured is the guy version, there's also a women's version that's like a modified bra.

On the subject of breathing, that is a big deal. You have to

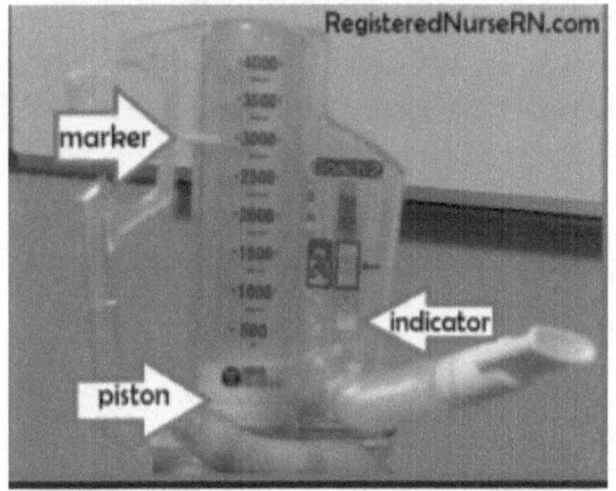

practice multiple times per hour with the "incentive spirometer". You suck in on the white tube and try to drive the piston up high on the marker. I was probably only able get to about to level 2250 in the hospital, while 3250 is normal for someone my age, but that improved quickly over time. This exercise is vital to keep your lungs clear and drive out any fluid from the pleural cavity. I didn't understand what the incentive was supposed to be, though. They didn't give me anything if I got my score higher. A lollipop for 2300 or ice cream for 2400 would have been nice.

It's in the step-down ward that you start doing PT, mostly short walks around the hallway that gradually get longer and longer. I was feeling pretty cocky doing that, when I had the stairway comeuppance I described in the beginning of the book. Stairs remained my nemesis for several months, although I got slowly better at them. It turned out the severity was worse in the early days because of continued fluid around the lungs.

I really had to adjust my attitude about rehab. I'd actually made a schedule before I'd gone into the hospital which had me riding my bike full tilt within 2 months, based on average rehab results I'd read about, and the smug notion "I'm an athlete, it'll go faster for me". That went right out the window. Time for baby steps. Try to be able to walk a little further each day, try to get a little better at stairs each day. And be grateful you're not in pain!

After my third night all my vitals were stable enough to send me home. There had been no signs of afib in the hospital and I was considered a relatively low stroke risk, so the only blood thinner I was on was baby aspirin. They took me off the strong diuretic (Lasix) and switched me to a weaker one, because the last chest x-ray in the hospital showed no fluid around the lungs. I had a repeat of the systemic reaction to surgery that I mentioned above about my first hip surgery. I'd also had a similar reaction after my second hip. I guess this is how my body complains when you put it through major trauma. This time the weird "antsy" feeling that interfered with sleep unfortunately lasted a couple of weeks. My blood pressure was abnormally low at this time so I could not get prescribed sleeping pills. It felt great when this finally went away.

My at-home instructions were to start walking 5 minutes a couple of times a day and ramp it up about a minute a day, And no lifting over 5 pounds (one of my precautions until the sternum healed). And I had to be really careful about not falling for the first couple of months while my sternum was vulnerable.

The sternal precautions can be summed up "Don't lift anything heavy, if it hurts don't do it, and don't fall". I was worried my upper body would atrophy by the time I was back to strength training, so after a couple of weeks I cobbled together a program of my own using the heart-hugger. I'd put it on, grab the handle with my left hand, tense my back and chest muscles, triceps and biceps, and do a benchpress motion with my right arm for about 12 reps. Then I'd switch hands, and do the exercise with my left. Then do left and right with a vertical press, again no weight, just tensed muscles fighting themselves. This caused no chest twinges of any sort and seemed to work pretty well.

I quickly got into a routine. I didn't work during this period. I read a lot and did my exercises and rehab, and we went on outings, like to restaurants or the store. It was great when I started walking outside (carefully, on nice flat sidewalks and paths). It was a bit amusing, though, when I ran into people I often had seen on my walks, usually brisk power walks with handweights. Now I was walking slowly and must have looked like I'd aged about 30 years. Don't worry, it's temporary, I'd assure them.

Having the goal of increasing my walks a bit each day helped me feel I was making progress, rather than focusing on how pitiful it seemed compared to my previous level of fitness.

Mental Aspects of Rehab

My routine kept me from having a problem that is very common after heart surgery: cardiac depression. Both Tilda and Adam mentioned getting it badly in their books. But they also both talked about laying around in the house in their bathrobes all day watching soap operas. I'd get depressed watching soap operas all day even without heart surgery. So-no moping around the house, get up, get dressed and get out every day, and move around as much as you can!

But up to 40% of patients get depression post-op, so there must be more to it than just the moping around and soap operas. It is more prevalent among people who have had a heart attack or stroke because it can be hard to trust your body again. Bob Harper, the famous trainer from "the Biggest Loser", had a near-fatal heart attack and described how psychologically challenging recovery was for him[61].

 Everybody is different, and this might be just another area where I was lucky. The at-home instructions from my surgeon mentioned depression and definitely recommended "get out every day", as well as how to get help if you're hit with depression.

The American heart association's website has some tips also. One suggestion both sources give is to take advantage of a structured cardiac rehab program when available, which is usually paid for by insurance. People who go through these programs have a much lower incidence of depression, and are also much less likely to have future cardiac incidents.

I think it helped a lot with my mental state that I practice mindfulness and meditation. Mindfulness is also known as "being in the present moment", something our society is unfortunately trending away from with everyone staring at their smartphones all day long. When you're going for a slow walk during rehab because that's all you can do right now, you can go along muttering "this sucks, I can't believe how slow I am, I wonder if I'll ever get better…" or you can pay attention to your surroundings and notice how nice the breeze on your face feels. For me, the latter is a lot more pleasant. Meditation is just sitting while focusing on something like your breath, which is great for stress relief and to avoid being fixated on negative trains of thought that can spiral into depression.

As I rehabbed, I enjoyed reading other people's stories of recovery for inspiration. <u>The Anna Meares Story</u> was great. She bounced back from breaking her neck in a track cycling sprint race accident to later win gold for Australia on the velodrome at the London Olympics. Another was <u>Iron Heart: The True Story of How I Came Back from the Dead</u>, by Brian Boyle. This young man recovered from a horrific accident when he was hit by a car on his bike, with massive internal injuries. Eventually, after rehab, he finished the Ironman triathlon in Hawaii.

These kind of stories illustrate that recovery is a long process requiring patience. It also does not always proceed on a predictable course of continued improvement, but is sometimes two steps forwards one step back, and you have to avoid getting discouraged by that. I tried to adopt that kind of mindset. Another recommendation I've read about to avoid depression is to set a physical goal for yourself that would indicate you were fully "back", like a marathon or ironman.

Having a goal sounds reasonable, but those seemed a bit extreme to me. I thought about it and realized there was a local combination bike-hike workout I liked: bike to the trailhead in Coyote Valley Open Space, hike the Arrowhead trail, bike back. This used to take me just over 2 hours before I'd started to have the heart valve symptoms. The last I had tried it, though, I got the out-of-breath symptom going up a steep section of trail that was like my heart announcing "ok, turn around, I'm done. Time to limp home with your tail between your legs". So I wrote down the goal that I would repeat this workout, in just over a couple of hours, as my goal after rehab.

Onward And (Mostly) Upward

After 10 days I had a follow-up with my surgeon's P.A. An x-ray of my back showed the pleural effusion had returned. That explained why I had been starting to feel more out of breath. The facility where I had my exam had more than one building, and I had to go to a different one for the x-ray, probably a few hundred feet away up a slight hill, but it took me forever to walk there. Another comedown from my former athletic glory! The fluid retention was so bad I had "cankles": there's so much swelling in your lower legs you can't see where your calves end and your ankles start. Also my feet were swelled. It felt weird to touch the flesh in this area, it was squishy. But the P.A. put me back on Lasix and the lungs quickly cleared up and the swelling went down. I lost 10 pounds of water weight in two days!

That may sound like a great weight loss program but it only works if there's so much water in your body it's hard to breathe and you think you're going to slosh when you walk. I had a second follow-up with the P.A. ten days later and everything looked ok. So they said they were done with me, wished me the best of luck, and said from now on I should follow up with my cardiologist.

I did have one other remaining symptom, my resting heart rate was still abnormally high. It was less than 60 before my surgery because I'm in decent shape, normal for my age is low to mid 70's. But mine was now in the 90s. This is common after open-heart surgery, a likely cause is pericarditis: the pericardium (membrane around the heart) can get inflamed because of surgical trauma. I was assured it would eventually clear up but could take up to a year.

I saw my surgeon for a follow-up at one month post-op. He showed me my ekg that indicated sinus rhythm (normal heart beat- no afib) and said "this means you aced the test". Karen said "no, you aced the test"! He said my body didn't know it had undergone surgery, it thought I'd been attacked by a mountain lion, so I had to give it time to heal and my resting heart rate would clear up. He said it would start to get better as I got my fitness back, and I was now cleared to go as hard as I wanted with cardio. I asked why I'd had such amazingly little sternal pain, was it he'd done such a good job on the sternal wiring? He laughed and said no, everybody is different. Other people might have lots of pain but not have the pleural effusion issue you had. It was wonderful talking to this great man who had saved my life.

Dr Gaudiani didn't have to tell me twice about doing harder cardio, I was chomping at the bit at this point. I still couldn't ride my bike or do my power walking with hand weights outside, so I joined the centennial rec center, a nice gym we have in Morgan Hill that's a collaboration between the city rec center and the Y. I'm not normally a fan of indoor exercise machines, but this was an exception- it felt great to be able to go hard again on machines like exercise bikes, the elliptical, and walking up a steep incline on the treadmill.

I followed up with my cardiologist a couple of weeks later. She thought my lungs didn't sound quite right and sent me for another x-ray. The effusion was back, perhaps not as bad as the previous episode but still serious.

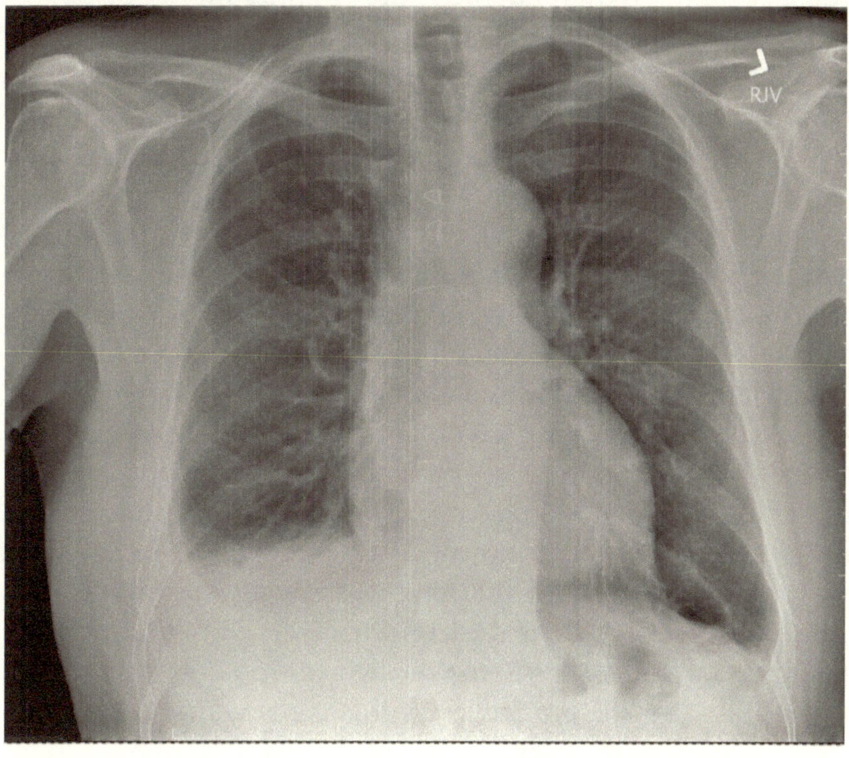

The black in the picture shows my lungs, expanded much smaller than they should be because of the fluid. If you look really close in the vicinity of the sternum you can see several of the wires that were put there to hold it together after surgery. They haven't caused any problem so there has been no need to take them out.

She put me back on the Lasix but said I'd stay on it until we were sure the fluid wasn't coming back. The effusion cleared up again in a few days. She also sent me for an echocardiogram, which showed the new valve functioning perfectly with a valve area back in the normal range. Because my original heart valve had been bicuspid, this valve area is probably higher than it had been in my entire life, so I was excited to see how it would perform when I recovered 100%. I was eventually able to get weaned off the Lasix, and thank goodness this time the pleural effusion hasn't come back (as of the time I'm writing, now well over a year post-op).

I felt good enough to start slowly going back to my freelance work at this time. Fortunately I work from home now and can set my own hours. When people tell me how lucky I am to be in this position, I remind them I paid my dues for decades commuting on US 101, which at one time had the honor of being named USA Today's worst commute in the country. My at-home instructions recommended starting cardiac rehab after 6 weeks. There is a nice rehab facility at El Camino so I gave them a call. I was concerned the level might be a little low for me, since my conditioning was already starting to improve. Julee, one of the directors, answered my questions and assured me they could make it as vigorous as I was ready for. The fact that she is an avid triathlete herself gave me even more confidence, so I signed up. My classes were to be Monday, Wednesday, Friday at 11 AM, which worked out fine because that is after rush hour trying to get from Morgan Hill to Mountain View.

But first I had to come in for an orientation session at 9:00 AM.
I decided to go up early before the brunt of rush hour and
sneak in a hike at a nearby open-space preserve beforehand.
Apparently that is not commonplace, when I arrived they
wanted me to do a six minute assessment walk to make sure I
was ready for rehab. But when I mentioned I'd come early and
done the hike they said "you went *hiking*? I think we can skip
the assessment".

I started rehab the next week and ended up going for 30
sessions. It was great. The staff was very nice and competent,
nurses and PTs specializing in cardiac rehab. The facility was
like a gym, but they had you wear a monitoring device that
was constantly checking your heart rate and for arrhythmias,
plus they would come by to get your blood pressure and see
how you were doing. I also could start using my arms on the
elliptical. I routinely ran my heart rate up to as much as 140
and we never saw arrhythmia in any of the sessions. And it
helped I could go hard with my arms on the machines without
bothering my sternum. Even though I couldn't do real
strength training yet I think the combination of this, and my
"heart hugger" strength routine described above, kept my
upper body from atrophying too badly. By the end of my 30
sessions, I was able to go quite strenuously without exceeding
my heart rate limit, and it was a great confidence booster
knowing that no heart abnormalities were detected.

I actually should have gone for 36 sessions except for a Medicare quirk. I hit 30 sessions at the end of December, and would be turning 65 in Jan, 2018, and be switching to Medicare. I could have had Medicare pay for the last 6 sessions, but they will only pay for one cardiac rehab stint per lifetime and I didn't want to waste it. I certainly hope to have no cardiac incidents to rehab from in the future, but one never knows. I thought that was a funny policy. "Didn't we pay for cardiac rehab for you a few years back? Shouldn't you be either better or dead by now?"

Around this time, after about 4 months post-op, my sternum was healed up enough to ride and hike (carefully!) outdoors, which I did on non-rehab days. It was really nice to be able to get back to working out outdoors again. I also was cleared to start strength training which I did in my garage gym, where I have dumbbells and exercise bands. You can get a good strength workout with bands as long as you use enough of them. They're not as nicely calibrated as weights, you can't say "I've added 5 pounds of weight since last week". Instead you get a qualitative sign of progress like "I replaced one of the red bands from last week with a stiffer blue band". The most important thing is you know you are progressing. I had to start with somewhat less resistance than before surgery, but over the next few months continued to get my strength back. I was also able to use hand weights while walking again without bothering my sternum, which felt great.

My neighbors seemed relieved to see me getting back to normal on my walks, or at least as close to normal as I get. I was also able stand up to pedal for long periods again, prior to this I'd quickly get out of breath. It was nice to have that activity back as I find in relaxing. I also started participating in group hikes again. At first I'd be lagging at the back of the group whenever the trail would get steep. My immediate goal was to be the second slowest so I could say "they're not having to wait up for me, it's that other guy". But over a few weeks my stamina came back and I was up at the front again. It felt like I was really getting somewhere when we climbed one of the biggest local peaks in the Santa Cruz Mountains, Mt. Umunhum, and I was able to keep up fine. That hike had over a thousand feet of vertical. But at the top of the trail there is a series of flights of stairs that I still lagged behind on. Stairs were still my nemesis!

My 65th birthday came in January 2018, about 5 ½ months post-op. By this time I was feeling great, able to all the activities I enjoy. I'm sure my performance was still a bit subpar but under the circumstances I didn't care. All in all, considering the seriousness of my condition and the major surgery I had undergone, I considered my recovery to date to be a nice birthday present and looked forward to continued improvement.

The only thing that persisted was the abnormally high resting heart rate. As Dr. Gaudiani had predicted, this improved a bit when I got fitter. But it was still in the 80s. It probably bugged me more than it should because I had always taken pride in a low resting heart rate being a sign that I was in good shape. I decided to get a second opinion on this so went to a different cardiologist. He did an ekg on me and it was normal. He said he was not concerned about the resting heart rate but we could drive it down by bumping up my dose of a beta-blocker, metoprolol, that I was already on, since I had no side effects from it. This lowered my resting heart rate into the low 70s and sometimes even the high 60s.

The best fix for my resting heart rate was when I stopped wearing my fitbit, which I had gotten before the surgery. I was getting kind of obsessive about it. Sitting at lunch, I'd peek and go "damn it, what's it doing back up in the 90s again?" Karen kept saying why don't you just take that thing off, but didn't get through to me. Then I mentioned to my brother that the high heart rate was my last symptom. He said, "so what, you said the doc isn't worried about it. Can you feel it thumping, does it keep you awake?" "No…" "How do you even know about it?" "I keep looking at my fitbit". "Why don't you just take the damn thing off?" "Oh…" Needless to say Karen rolled her eyes when I told her "Bill gave me a great idea", but she was still happy I took it off. No offense to fitbit, activity trackers can be great as long as you don't obsess over them.

In March I redid my goal workout, the Arrowhead loop, in 2 hours and 7 minutes. I blitzed right up the section of trail where I had gotten badly out of breath when my aortic stenosis was bad. So it was great to be able to say "I'm Baaack"! This was at seven months postop. Update at about a year and a quarter post-op: I repeated the Mt. Umunhum hike the other day, and was delighted to be able to briskly motor right up the stairs at the end, and I also recently broke 2 hours on the Arrowhead loop, a new PR. And my resting heart rate is back down to 60. Considering the severity of the condition that had gotten fixed and how much tougher this rehab turned out to be than I anticipated, that's not bad at all.

It's really nice to be fit and healthy again instead of the sorry state I'd probably be in by now if I hadn't gotten this fixed. In my old age adventures so far, I got two new hips for my 60th birthday, and a new heart valve for my 65th. Karen says she'd really rather I didn't get any replacement parts for my 70th. I'm inclined to agree with her.

My Activity Now

I do a combination of hiking and biking, with occasional cross-country skiing in the winter and kayaking or stand-up paddling in warmer months. I also do "heavyhands" walking with hand weights, which I describe in chapter 3. I have a garage gym with dumbbells and bands. It feels good that in addition to gaining back any strength and muscle mass I lost post-surgery, I'm a lot stronger than when I first set up this gym almost 10 years ago. At this age the "inevitable decline with age" was supposed to make me lose muscle mass, and should have been worse because of the speedbump I went through with the heart valve surgery.

I do what's called "polarized" training (described in chapter 3). On a hard day, maybe twice a week, I do full body resistance workouts, and high intensity interval training for both lower and upper body. These sessions are shorter but intense. Sometimes I also throw in some longer less intense intervals to work on improving my "cruising speed". The next day is an easy day. On the other days I bike and/or hike at a brisk but comfortable pace, with longer days a couple of times a week. The hikes are often with friends (part of my social support).

Every night I do a yoga routine that I've cobbled together from classes I've taken and books I've read over the years. Great for stress management and to keep me limber, which gets more important with age. At 65 I'm as flexible as when I was 30.

Lately I discovered a cool medicare benefit for us old folks: *Silver Sneakers*. You can get free memberships in participating gyms, so now I added going to my local 24 hour fitness to the mix. I take yoga classes there, and supplement my home strength training with their equipment. Though I prefer outdoors, the gym is a nice bad weather option also. That's my formal activity. Throughout the day I always try to keep moving and not sit too long. I have a timer that pops up on my computer to remind me to do some moving.

What It's Like To Enjoy Exercise

Physical activity is not a "pill" that I take because it's good for me or to lose weight. After I got to where I could do endurance activities like biking, hiking, running, or walking consistently for sessions longer than about 30 minutes, they became enjoyable, something I looked forward to, instead of a chore. I describe in chapter 2 what can be done to make this be true for a lot of people.

My main activities, biking and hiking, and occasional paddling, are now my hobbies. I love planning them, "my group is hiking Skyline Ridge next Saturday that looks fun" or "I haven't biked Coyote Creek to Hellyer Park and back recently, Sunday would be a nice day for that". It's also nice to have longer term goals to point towards, like: "Senior games time trial coming up in the spring, better start throwing in some more longer intervals to bump up my speed". In addition I like to also read inspirational stories about athletes, and other people who have rehabbed from illness of injury and bounced back to do something challenging. All of this is a lot more fun than taking a pill! Or sitting in a rocking chair, which used to be considered a more appropriate activity at my age.

Chapter 2- Fitness Motivation: Making it Enjoyable

We are not meant to be sedentary. It is only starting in the 20th century, with the rise of automobiles and desk jobs, that it even became possible for anyone but the wealthiest to be "couch potatoes". The physical activity of early European settlers in Australia, for example, was estimated to exceed that of their modern counterparts by the equivalent of 16 km of walking per day (10 miles)[33]. Amish farmers in the Appalachian part of Ohio, who live a traditional non-mechanized lifestyle, walk the equivalent of at least 9 miles a day and on top of that do a lot more high intensity activity than non-Amish in the same region[75].

There are well-known detrimental health effects of a sedentary lifestyle, and the combination of inactivity and poor diet is especially harmful. Obesity is strongly correlated with physical inactivity[67]. It can become a vicious circle, the more overweight you get, the less you feel like moving. Most adults in the Western world do not get enough physical activity, and only 10% of the people over age 60 exercise regularly. I discuss the important topic "physical activity, health, and longevity" in the appendix.

That was originally going to be the subject of this chapter, because I figured that explaining all the various ways being active prevents declines with aging and promotes health would be the best motivation. Then I read <u>No Sweat: How The Simple Science Of Motivation Can Bring You A Lifetime Of Fitness</u>, by Dr. Michelle Segar, whose work is specifically on the subject of motivating people to be active. She points out that exercising for an external reason, like losing weight or health benefits, makes people view it as a chore rather than something enjoyable. That is perhaps why 67% of the gym ownerships in the US are not used[139]. People join because they know it's something they "should" be doing, force themselves to go for a while, then get tired of "taking the pill". Same thing for all the exercise equipment in homes or garages with cobwebs on it.

It is important to have the "right why" to exercise, according to Dr. Segar (and she gives plenty of evidence in her excellent book to back it up). What is needed is an internal reward, like moving because it is fun or relaxing. I am fortunate enough to have found ways of being active that I enjoy. I look forward to it, and feel more relaxed after doing it. So if you're not currently physically active, the top priority is for you to find something for yourself to enjoy. Exercising because you like it, because it will relax you, you'll feel better after, it will clear your brain, etc., are all examples of the right why: internal motivation. Exercising to lose weight, lower your blood pressure, live longer, are all external.

Now imagine you've set your alarm a half hour earlier to fit a nice walk in to start your day. The alarm rings and the argument in your head starts.

- Version 1- "Who needs a walk, I want to sleep another half hour" "But remember this will make us live longer" "Who cares? I don't want to live longer if it means you're going to get me up at the crack of dawn every damn day".
- Version 2- "Who needs a walk, I want to sleep another half hour". "We had this conversation yesterday. You were cranky about getting up but remember how much better you felt afterwards." "I'm still cranky. Oh all right I'll get up".

Version 2, based on internal motivation, is more likely to succeed in the long run. One attitude problem that prevent many of us from enjoying being active is the notion that exercise has to be vigorous enough to work up a sweat, or last a long enough amount of time, to "count"[139]. But there's more and more evidence that accumulating small bouts of movement throughout the day is health promoting. Taking several short walks per day is a lot better than sitting all day.

How Much and What Type?

Before I get to ways to make exercise enjoyable, it's important to discuss how much activity is currently recommended and what is the best type. Typically you'll see recommendations like 2½ hours total per week, or "30 minutes per day on most days". These guidelines are often too generic in that they don't distinguish between cardio and resistance training, or low and high intensity training.

It turns out, as shown in the appendix, that there is pretty strong evidence that resistance training and higher intensity cardio (also called high intensity interval training, or HIIT) give the most "bang for the time buck" for anti-aging and metabolic benefits. These can be done in as little as two 30 minute sessions per week on non-consecutive days. That can be supplemented with just moving around more and sitting less on other days, and may be a lot easier to fit into your schedule than 2½ hours. If you don't enjoy exercise and think of it as "taking a pill", at least this is a smaller pill to swallow.

But don't be too quick to assume that you won't enjoy higher intensity. Look at kids at the playground, they often run around in short bursts, they're not continuously jogging. Or a dog chasing a ball, that's a full on sprint. And dogs don't look like they think it's a chore. My brother had a great dog, Pete, a lab/border collie mix. I was throwing a ball for him, it seemed like a hundred times or so, until Bill said "you realize, he'll keep doing that until either he collapses or your arm falls off". Working up to a fast pace can feel great, like how I imagine it must feel for a frisky colt stretching its legs. I especially enjoy doing HIIT if I'm at a gym, which I find less enjoyable than outdoors. A short 30 minute workout with high intensity thrown in goes by quickly and leaves me feeling energized.

Sneaking in Some NEAT

Physical activity does not mean just exercise. The latest word is NEAT (non-exercise activity thermogenesis), with the catchphrase "sitting is the new smoking"[27, 82].

Dr. James Levine describes this in detail in his book <u>Get Up!: Why Your Chair is Killing You and What You Can Do About It</u>.[83] I remember seeing a fun British documentary (BBC's "The truth about exercise" by Michael Mosley), where the 24 hour energy expenditure was measured for a waitress in a café compared to a very fit looking young man who worked out hard in the gym but had a desk job. Her 24 hour energy burn beat his hands down, with her chart showing constant movement all day long, while his showed low activity except one spike during his time at the gym.

So the first thing to work on is bumping up NEAT, moving throughout the day and avoiding sitting for too long. I do this with a timer on my computer that pops up every 20 minutes to remind me to get out of the chair and move around. It can seem to do this at inopportune times, but it is worth it to me. Activity trackers on smartphones and watches can do the same thing. I witnessed an amusing example of this the other day after a group hike, when we went to lunch. A friend was wearing a Fitbit and it vibrated, the little guy started dancing, and it said "you've been sitting for 20 minutes. Time to move!". She said "I just hiked for 3 hours. Cut me a break!" There is lots of advice around on how physical activity can be sprinkled throughout the day, by doing things like parking further away, using the stairs instead of the elevator, etc. Stairs are especially good because they provide a bit of higher intensity activity which we normally don't get in daily living.

The problem with this approach is that people can dabble at it and not have any idea how much activity they are doing. This was first addressed with pedometers and the 10,000 steps guideline, which, I just found out from good old Wikipedia, originated in Japan in 1965[172]. There's nothing magic about exactly 10,000 steps. I think the important thing is first just wear the pedometer (or fitness tracker) all day and audit what your steps are for a typical day, then set a goal to bump that up over time.

I believe that using fitness trackers in this manner is one of their best applications. And it's better not to be constantly looking at them while active, it takes away from mindfulness, which we'll discuss in chapter 5. Check out the data later, nerding out on all the graphs you want. Just remember that the accuracy of some of the measurements, plus the formulae used to make some of the estimates, is questionable. For example using a fitness tracker to estimate "calories burned" is not particularly accurate.

Active Transportation

I'm also a fan of active transportation, like walking, biking, roller blading, etc., to commute or do errands. In the US and some other modern countries, many of our cities had become too car-centric and not walk- or bike-friendly, but thankfully that trend seems to be reversing.

There is a really cool Ted talk ("How an obese town lost a million pounds") by Mick Cornett, the mayor of Oklahoma City, on how Oklahoma City got itself off the list of 50 "fattest" towns in the US and moved it onto the list of 50 "fittest" towns by getting more active, which required various changes to make it more walkable[191]. This also had the side effect of attracting more young talented professionals to work in the city, and OKC now has one of the strongest economies in the US. As well as a great basketball team.

There is a detailed discussion of the benefits of active transportation in general and cycling in particular in Peter Walker's How Cycling Can Save the World. For a significant increase in active transportation there has to be enough spending on infrastructure so people feel safe doing it. We already saw how that worked out for Oklahoma city, and the most famous examples are countries like Holland and Denmark where as 30% or more of trips are by bike. In Utrecht, Holland, it is an astonishing 60%. The coolest tidbit from the book was about aging people who can no longer drive safely. That is a sad loss of freedom and mobility in people's lives. But less so in Holland, where the just go back to biking, and with the advent of electric pedal-assist, are doing so into their 80s.

Bikenomics: How Bicycling Can Save The Economy by Elly Blue describes how incredibly cost effective it is to invest in active transportation infrastructure, compared to roads or even mass transportation. Motorists often have the objection that they are subsidizing other forms of transportation with their vehicle fees and gas taxes. Elly shows that this is not the case, that it is roads themselves that are subsidized: local roads are only about 10% funded by vehicle fees and gas taxes, and free parking is also a big subsidy.

Another concern is that bike infrastructure will interfere with motorized traffic but properly planned projects can often improve traffic flow[216]. Here's an obvious example: parallel parking in a crowded downtown holds up car traffic for two reasons. First a lane is blocked while someone is backing into a space. Second, a significant amount of traffic in a downtown is people driving around looking for a parking space. So a win-win project is to remove the on-street spaces and replace them with a parking garage. The width formerly taken up by on-street parking can accommodate a protected bike lane and some landscaping or a wider sidewalk.

I discovered active transportation when I commuted by bike. There's nothing more motivating than having your activity be the fastest way to get somewhere. "Exercise? I don't have time" is no longer an excuse when it's actually saving you time. I still do lots of errands on my bike. And when I go to the gym by bike, rather than getting to and from the gym making the workout more time consuming, it's part of the workout.

Another obvious example of sneaking exercise in is walking the dog. I've only once personally witnessed the sad sight of someone driving slowly down the road with their door open and a leash hanging out with Fido trotting along. More often I'll see people on bikes slowly pedaling while the dog walks. Forget the car and the bike, enjoy the outdoors, on foot, with your dog.

These are all a great start for someone who does not like to exercise. Dr. Segar also devotes a chapter "from a chore to a gift" on how to convert exercise from something you "should" do to a gift to yourself of something you enjoy, like play time was when we were kids. You may have to experiment with a few activities to find one that's enjoyable. Below are some suggestions from my experience.

Delayed gratification

Exercise can certainly be enjoyable, but not necessarily right away. Like jumping into the swimming pool on a hot day, it's great once you're in, but you can be hesitant to take the plunge. If you're trying to fit your workout in first thing in the morning and have to get up earlier to do that, it's going to seem like a much better idea to hit the snooze button. Nike had a great commercial illustrating this. A woman is sitting on the side of her bed, bleary-eyed, and the bed starts talking to her in seductive tones- "You want me. You know you want me. I am so warm, so comfortable...". She shakes off the siren call, grabs her running shoes and leaves. If you are able to be disciplined like her, and just get going you'll feel better afterwards and all day. If you get in the habit of doing this consistently, it gets easier to fight off the little voice of temptation.

Effortless, not "no pain, no gain"

"No pain, no gain" is the first thing that has to go from the "it doesn't count" mentality. Even strolling at a "museum walk" pace is better than sitting. But for me, a brisker but still pleasant pace is the most relaxing. It should feel like you could keep it up all day. The "talk test" is a classic way to tell pace. You should be able to carry on a conversation while doing the activity. If you feel somewhat out of breath it's too fast. There's nothing wrong with going fast if you enjoy it, as some people do, but many find a more comfortable pace more relaxing.

As for "no pain, no gain", with the effortless pace you'll be pleasantly surprised, if you do it consistently, that after a few weeks you've "gained" quite a bit. You'll now be able to go a lot farther, and you may notice that the pace that feels comfortable now is faster than it was a few weeks ago.

But what if I'm trying to lose weight? Won't I burn a lot less calories at a comfortable pace than if I push myself? This is a point Dr. Segar talks about a lot in her book. Here are two scenarios (which come from an actual case study of one of her clients). In the first you're fired up with your New Year's resolution, work out hard, get burned out after 3 weeks, and give up. In the second, you do something you enjoy at a comfortable pace, and are able to keep it going consistently. You'll burn a lot more calories the second way in a year, than the first way of 3 hard weeks followed by 49 weeks of sitting.

But most importantly, as I discuss in chapter 4, calorie burn is not the most vital aspect of physical activity for weight loss. Aside from various other health benefits of moving, specifically it has metabolic effects like lowering insulin resistance that help with weight loss. And many of these benefits happen at a comfortable pace.

Or- Go Harder for Shorter

An alternative to the comfortable paced approach is to do higher intensity activities for a shorter amount of time. Dr. Martin Gibala and colleagues have done pioneering research in this area. It's been known for some time that high intensity interval training is a good way to build fitness in brief sessions. But most training protocols used in studies were really hard, like repeating hard 4 minute intervals 4 times. Speaking from experience, those can hurt towards the end.

Dr. Gibala worked on finding interval training for those of us that wanted a short brisk workout without a lot of discomfort. He's experimented with it for many years and finally came up with 3x20 seconds (shorthand for go hard for 20 seconds, recover at an easy pace, and repeat 3 times). He calls this "the one minute workout" because the hard part is only for a minute. The whole workout is actually 10 minutes with warmup and cooldown. Doing this just 3 times a week confers good health benefits[50].

As an example of the intense part, you could climb briskly upstairs for 20 seconds, then walk slowly down, and repeat 3 times. Or if you live in a two story house, you could just go briskly up and down the stairs, and keep doing it for one minute (with a warmup before and cooldown after).

The idea originally was to come up with a short session for people who don't like to exercise to "get it over with". But surprisingly it's been found that many people enjoy this type of workout more. The intervals break up any monotony, and 20 seconds is long enough to be challenging at a higher intensity but not long enough to be too uncomfortable.

I do intervals a couple of times a week, and enjoy the short brisk session that leaves me feeling exhilarated afterwards. But I emphasize Dr. Segar's point that physical activity at a comfortable pace "counts" just as much, just do whichever you like more. If you're interested in the "short and sweet" approach I recommend Dr. Gibala's book <u>The One Minute Workout</u>.

Resistance training can also be done in a short time by sticking to a single set of relatively few exercises that cover major muscle groups. You can combine resistance training and interval training on the same day, and pretty readily fit both into a 30 minute session, with a warmup, followed by a short interval session, the resistance session, and a cooldown. And since we need recovery after high intensity training, especially as we get older, these should be done only a couple of times a week, on non-consecutive days, with easy (comfortably paced) days or days off in between.

Meditation in motion

Any kind of repetitive activity like walking, running, biking, skating, canoeing, kayaking, swimming, etc., can spontaneously get you into a relaxed meditative state. I talk about meditation specifically in chapter 5, but here I'm referring to letting the relaxation happen by itself by noticing the rhythm of the breath or your footfalls (or cycling cadence, paddle strokes, etc.), or both together.

Hopefully you can also find a nice place to do this, like a park or trail, and get natural relaxation from the scenery. The effortless pace is conducive to the "meditative" feeling. Needless to say, you will not get this feeling if you are fussing with your phone during the activity.

Valid Thoughts And "The Gate At 5 Miles"

When you are first starting an exercise program, you will encounter a lot of mental resistance that I alluded to in the "argument with yourself" above. It helps to keep in mind that this is just mental noise no matter how valid the reasoning seems to you at the time, and will go away if you keep going long enough. When I was going on long runs or bike rides, I'd often notice that I'd feel great once I got into the workout and afterwards I would be nice and mellow and be glad I had gone.

But I would still get the negative mental chatter when starting out: "this is BS. I ran yesterday. Why do I have to run every day. You're making me run 6 miles are you crazy? I could go on a reasonable run, like 2 miles! Then I could have slept in another half hour". Finally I came up with the rule that my thoughts weren't valid until I'd been going at least 15 minutes or so. So during the initial negative period I'd just observe the negativity and think "yeah, whatever". After about 15 minutes the chatter would die down and I'd get the pleasant, flowing, meditation-in-motion feeling. Now that I practice mindfulness, described in chapter 5, I can just observe negative thoughts that arise and not get caught up in them. And the chatter seems to go away more quickly.

The other thing is that it gets easier after you become fit enough to do an endurance activity like walking, hiking, running, or biking for at least 30 minutes continuously. I remember reading a book about running where the author introduced the term "the gate at 5 miles". He said if he asked people who ran why they did it, those who averaged less than 5 miles on their runs would usually answer something like "I'm trying to lose weight" or "I'm trying to stay healthy". Those who averaged more than 5 miles would say something more like "because I enjoy it".

This rule of thumb was certainly true for me. I think this generalizes to all endurance activities. The transition from it being something that you are doing because you "should", to something you do because you enjoy it, starts to occur naturally after you can go consistently for more than 30 minutes or so.

Making Some Specific Activities Enjoyable

Walking

This is the most natural activity for most people, since it's just an extension of an activity of daily living. Just try to sneak it in as often as possible. In rainy weather get a nice big umbrella, in cold weather wear a scarf or ski mask in necessary. When I lived in Boulder we once had a cold snap of -20° F for a couple of weeks. I walked and ran during that period wearing a balaclava and a surgeon's mask to warm up my breath. It was challenging at first but exhilarating afterwards. Saner people than me can always find indoor places to walk in such conditions.

Walking is one of the best ways to get the meditative feeling I mentioned. Your arm swing, gait, and breathing all fall into harmony and you notice your surroundings. Being in a beautiful outdoor place obviously helps.

If I had to pick a single activity to do, it would probably be walking. When rehabbing from my heart valve replacement, building up to where I could walk again at a decent pace for a longer period was my most important goal. I would have felt great if that was all I had been able to get back to.

Another benefit of walking is that the activity feels enjoyable and natural right away for many people. For running you have to build up to it, using run-walk transition programs as described in chapter 3. It may not be comfortable at first, but will feel better after a few weeks. For biking there are comfort issues that will resolve when, for example, your butt toughens up. But it may not feel great until then. But lots of people can go for a 5 minute walk and feel good right away. You then can just add a minute a day or so, enjoying the activity the whole time, and get to the "gate at 30 minutes" described above in a few weeks.

As you get fitter you can start making your pace a bit brisker. Or look for some places nearby to hike. You can always try transitioning to running later if you feel like it, and it should be easier than starting from scratch.

A variation on walking is to carry hand weights. I'll describe more about the technique in the next chapter. I actually find that this can add to the enjoyment, the weights make me feel the rhythm of the "four-limbed" motion more. Try walking with a vigorous arm swing using the weights and see if you enjoy it.

If not, forget about it. To paraphrase what Mark Twain said about golf, I wouldn't want hand weights to cause a good walk to be spoiled. There's one caveat I'd like to mention about walking specifically: a lot of books teach "power walking" with arms bent unnaturally at 90 degrees. That actually comes from race walking, where it makes sense because you're going so fast that a natural arm swing has trouble keeping up with your gait. At slower than race pace, though, it actually makes it a less vigorous exercise, as well as ruining the natural feel of the walk.

Hiking

Walking gets a bit more challenging when you take it on trails, especially uphill, but the trails are often in beautiful settings. I like to use hiking poles because it keeps some of the impact from my hips when going downhill. It also makes me, a naturally clumsy person and prone to ankle sprains in my youth, more sure-footed.

Hiking is great with a group. If you don't have friends that like to hike, you can find good groups on www.meetup.com. Hiking is a good choice for noncompetitive people because you can still challenge yourself to get stronger. The reward is being able to go places where you couldn't otherwise be able to, earning yourself some killer views in the process.

The views from the north rim of the Grand Canyon, Longs Peak, Mount Missouri, Half-done, Mt. Tallac, and other places are very fond memories for me. But at 65 I am not just looking back. There are lots of challenges in my local area and beyond that still await. Recent views from the Pinnacles, Mt. Umunhum, and Sentinel Dome in Yosemite rank right up there with any from the past, and that's just scratching the surface of what I'd like to do. I take to heart the advice I read somewhere recently: "never let your dreams get smaller than your memories".

Running

I think a lot of us have kind of a love-hate relationship with running. On the one hand we may remember joyously doing it as kids, just running around playing. But we also may have learned along the way to think of it as a chore or punishment, like when you mess up in practice and the coach tells you to "go take a lap". In fact I've seen runners wearing t-shirts "my sport is your sport's punishment".

I think people who enjoy running are able to get back to the fun feeling from being a kid. And it also helps to keep the pace comfortable. Running was the first activity that caused me to get into the spontaneous meditative state mentioned above, the footfalls and breath just came together naturally long before I'd read about any of those concepts. Once you get to enjoy running itself, trail running becomes another option. There's a lot of overlap with hiking, like getting away from it all in great scenery. With trail running you can cover more ground and see even more scenery. And after you've earned it by a big uphill climb, running downhill is a quicker way to get back down as well as being fun.

Biking

Here's another activity that takes us back to being kids. The feeling when you were first able to ride a bike on your own, and the freedom of how far you could go under your own power. A lot of our cities our getting more bike friendly now, with good bike lanes or car-free bikepaths. If you're afraid of traffic you can find a safe route through proper planning that combines quiet residential streets and streets with good bike lane.

Or you can always throw the bike in a trunk or on a bike rack and take it to the trailhead of a bikepath. The other obstacle can be comfort. I discuss ways to deal with that in the next chapter.

An interesting variation of biking is standing up to pedal using a higher gear. This is more comfortable, a great workout, and feels more like running (but impact-free). There are special running bikes like the Elliptigo that more closely mimic running, which some people swear by. Personally I find standup pedaling on a regular bike just as enjoyable. Top gear on my trek hybrid is about 120 inches, which is more than enough. My superpro has a top gear of 91 which is a bit brisk for standing but I still enjoy it. Gear inches are described in the appendix.

Paddling

Canoeing, stand-up, and kayak paddling are fun activities that are a great upper body workout. I'd recommend lessons because novices tend to just "arm paddle" which is exhausting and not fun. Proper canoe and stand-up paddling involves leaning forward with the torso and then pulling back so you're using your back muscles as well as arms, while kayak paddling involves your oblique muscles in a torso twist. Once you get the hang of it, these are both smooth relaxing movements. And you can sure get to some nice places on the water.

Dancing

Some people enjoy aerobic dance classes but to others this smacks too much of "exercise". Nowadays there are more fun alternatives like Zumba, with good music and in a friendly social atmosphere. I haven't tried them but I know people who swear by them. Gyms and City Rec centers or adult ed often have classes like these or good old fashioned ballroom dancing, line dancing, etc.

Exercise Classes At Gyms

Classes offer another way to get some fellowship and make exercise fun. There are a ton of different classes available nowadays such as boot camp, functional fitness, pilates, tai chi, trx, yoga, and zumba.

Crossfit

Crossfit is an amazing alternative to conventional gyms, with good camaraderie and everyone cheering each other on during workouts. If you have watched the Crossfit games, crowning what Crossfit has a very strong claim to being the fittest men and women on earth, you might get scared off by the astonishing displays of strength and endurance. But those are world-class athletes, what you'd be doing at your local Crossfit is more attainable, and they have the concept of "scaled WODs": for example, the workout of the day (WOD), might call for squats with a heavy weighted barbell, but you would start out with a PVC pipe and work yourself up to the barbell over time.

Sports

For many people, participating in sports like golf, tennis, basketball, softball, flag football, is the most fun way to get in a workout. Pickleball is starting to be popular now, with a lot of the fun of tennis but less skill required. You can also get a good workout from table tennis, which Dr. Daniel Amen refers to as the best brain workout[197]. I've been thinking of getting back into that, I was pretty good at it in my youth, but I'd have to park my ego at the door- Our rec center in Morgan Hill has people older than me that would give me a serious thrashing.

Running and biking also have their competitive versions. For biking I recommend time trials more than road races, as the folks I know that participate in road racing have all crashed from time to time. Many of these sports can qualify as higher intensity as well. And they can motivate you to do resistance training to get better at your sport.

My only concern is that you develop your muscles symmetrically. I remember a couple of avid golfers who worked out at the gym I used to go to. They'd spend a lot of time doing a torso twist station to improve their drive. But they'd only do it in one direction. I figured they had well-developed oblique muscles on one side, and atrophy on the other.

None of the above?

There are various other alternatives if none of the above are appealing. Roller blading was a lot of fun for me (in between falls). The motion itself is fun when you can get a good rhythmic glide going. Cross country skiing, including roller skiing, has a similar feel. There's the "kick and glide" of classic skiing, or skate skiing which feels similar to roller blading, but at least for me is safer (if I stay on easy terrain) because snow is softer to fall on than concrete or asphalt! The kick scooters kids use with the steering handles come in adult versions. They look like a lot of fun, and a good quick way of getting around. My wife won't let me try one. She's taken me to the hospital one too many times. But if I were younger and less clumsy maybe…

You may need to be adaptable if life throws you a curve and you can no longer do your favorite activity, as when I could no longer run due to arthritis. Around that time I would read avid lifetime runners saying they didn't know what they would do if they could no longer run. Well, I just found enjoyment in bicycling instead. Then I read an enthusiastic bicyclist saying "I'll keep bicycling until I can no longer throw a leg over the top tube". Uh, I already can't do that- my hips are too stiff. So I would lay the bike down, step over the tube, and pick it back up (fortunately no longer necessary with my new hips). When I watched the 2018 Paralympic winter games on TV from PyeongChang, Korea, I witnessed lots of people who have worked around more difficult limitations than me.

But maybe not everybody finds an activity they like so much they want to set aside time for it in longer continuous stretches. Remember there's always activities of daily living to fall back on. If you can keep from sitting too long at a stretch, and move more throughout the day, you'll be a lot healthier than someone who sits all day, as described in <u>Get Up!: Why Your Chair is Killing You and What You Can Do About It</u>. Hopefully these interludes of activity will start to be enjoyable breaks in your routine that you look forward to.

Stephen Guise's book <u>Mini Habits: Smaller Habits, Bigger Results</u> shows how to start phasing physical activity in slowly for those who don't enjoy it and/or are having trouble getting started. He gives the fascinating example of how he made the simple change of doing 1 pushup a day, on a regular basis. On some days he'd feel enthused and do more, and maybe throw in some other physical activity afterwards, on others he'd just do the minimum, but he never missed a day. This gradually led to him enjoying exercise, which he now does on a regular basis.

Making Resistance Training Enjoyable

Most of the activities I've described so far contribute to aerobic conditioning. It is important to also supplement that with resistance training to prevent loss of muscle and bone mass with age (described in the appendix). You could optionally not worry about this until you're well established in an activity you like that keeps you moving on a regular basis.

My Uncle Din walked vigorously until he died at 92, and
didn't fade until a few months from the end. That was pretty
much all he did, except for any upper body activity he got
from daily life. He did get slower, and frail in the upper body.
But he could do all his activities of daily living just fine.

If you do want to supplement with some upper body work,
it's much better if you can make that enjoyable too. Doing
swimming, heavyhands, Nordic walking, paddling, or cross
country skiing are all helpful. Otherwise you may need to
throw in some resistance training.

In the next chapter I'll describe a simple workout with 5
movements, 1 set each, which covers the upper body well,
including the core, in only a few minutes. I find it enjoyable if
I do these slowly and mindfully, it's almost like the feeling of
doing yoga. It also helps motivate me that there are other
activities like cross country skiing and paddling that these
keep me in better shape for.

Chapter 3-Physical Training Tips For Health And Fighting Off The "Inevitable" Declines With Aging

There are three areas where our bodies decline with age: aerobic capacity, muscles, and higher intensity capabilities. How these affect health is described in detail in the appendix. Also, sitting too much is not healthy in its own right. So the most important thing is to fit in ways to keep moving throughout the day, or adding NEAT to your daily activities, as we saw in chapter 2. If you do enough of that it also serves as your aerobics workout, occurring throughout the day rather than in a single dedicated session. If you're currently mostly sedentary, that means the top priority is to find an activity you enjoy such as walking that you can fit in throughout the day. If you find an activity you really like, as I have been fortunate enough to do, it's likely you'll look forward to setting aside time for dedicated sessions because you feel better and more relaxed afterwards. It's amazing what a nice brisk 30 minute walk, run, bike ride or (fill in your favorite) does for your state of mind. When you are well established in consistent daily movement, and are wondering, "this is great, what next?", it's also important to consider the other two aspects, resistance training and higher intensity.

Resistance Training- If it's not your favorite

For people who don't really enjoy doing resistance training, and just want to hang on to muscle mass, I'm going to describe a short program that hits the high notes. If you like strength training, bear with me, we'll get to that next. For the purposes of maintaining muscle mass with age and other health benefits of resistance training, a single set of each exercise is sufficient, as recommended by the American College of Sports Medicine[192]. It is controversial whether more sets are needed for other purposes such as optimally building muscle mass, but one set is fine for health. The minimum movements for the upper body are a horizontal pull (like a rowing machine), a horizontal push (like pushups or benchpress), a vertical pull (like pullups or a pulldown machine), a vertical push (the vertical press), an abdominal movement like crunches, and a back strengthener like the "good morning" exercise (bowing from the waist and straightening up). One set of 8 reps is a good start. The resistance should be high enough that getting to 8 is challenging. Add more reps as they get easier, when you get to 12 you should add more resistance and drop back to 8 reps[192]. The equipment or free weights to do these are found in any gym. Or you can do them at home:
- The pushes are easy with minimal equipment,
  - Just the floor for pushups (from the knees when just starting out, from the feet with straight legs when you get stronger). Or you can use a bench to do bench presses with dumbbells, or even lie on your back on the floor and do bench presses with dumbbells with a slightly restricted range of motion.
  - The vertical push can be done seated or standing with dumbbells.

- Pullups can be done with a pullup bar (you can get one that hangs from a doorway). If you are not strong enough yet, you can use pullup assist bands, and gradually reduce the amount of assist as you get stronger. Alternatively you can use resistance bands attached to an eye bolt in a stud high on a wall (mine are in the garage) to do a pulldown.
- Resistance bands also work great, mounted lower on the wall, for the rowing motion. Or you can do one side at a time with dumbbells: get on all fours and make the rowing motion with the dumbbell in your right hand, then switch sides.
- An alternative to crunches and "good mornings", that also provides a leg and arm workout, is double poling with weights and/or resistance bands, discussed below under heavyhands.

All of the above can be completed in less than 10 minutes if you stick to one set (which is plenty for general health)[192], and twice a week should be plenty. This is the "taking a pill version" of resistance training, but at least the pill is as small as possible. An alternative is to break it up as part of your NEAT. As I recommended in chapter 2, it's a good idea to have a timer remind you to take a break from sitting once in a while. A couple of days a week, when you get some of your reminders, instead of going for a walk, do a resistance movement. Another approach to resistance training is to try to make it fun by taking a group class. My local "Y" has a "functional fitness for 50+" class that uses weights with '50s music. Or, as I mentioned in the previous chapter, you can get upper body training in activities like heavyhands (described in more detail below), Nordic walking, cross country skiing, paddling, or swimming. You can also use exercise machines like ellipticals with arms, or the Schwinn Airdyne or Rogue Assault Airbike with arm action. You really also need a squat or leg press type movement to keep your legs strong. I omitted that because you can accomplish the same thing as part of your higher intensity training, such as going fast up stairs, discussed below. I get a good "fast twitch muscle fiber" workout for my legs with "on-bike strength training" (pedaling uphill in a high gear), and sprint training on my bike. Now that I have access to a gym through "silver sneakers", I also do single leg presses with the leg press machine. This is not to brag but to demonstrate that the on-bike strength training must have been effective, because that was all I had been doing for leg strength for years: when I first returned to the gym I could do the full weight stack (400 lbs.) when using both legs on that machine. I had to go to single leg presses to make it challenging.

Resistance Training- If You Like It

If you like resistance training, then I'm going to assume you know plenty about it and you don't need any advice on technique, sets, and reps. But an important issue that arises is that lots of people that like resistance training don't like aerobics. The good news is you don't have to do any. I'd still recommend NEAT breaks to avoid sitting too much, and other ways to sneak activity into activities of daily living like stairs instead of elevators. That is already providing some aerobics. But you can also kill three birds with one stone doing resistance training, if you do it as high intensity interval training. It is then a combination of resistance training, high intensity training, and aerobics, in one highly time efficient package. Circuit training was probably the earliest version of this. Early studies showed this did not have enough cardio benefits, but that was because it was not done at a high enough intensity. A similar type of training has recently been made famous by CrossFit, they call it "metcon" (short for metabolic conditioning). And no one can accuse Crossfitters of not working out with enough intensity.

Higher Intensity Training

Higher intensity training is important for several reasons as shown in the appendix. For example, the ability to exercise at higher intensity corresponds with longevity, and higher intensity training has important metabolic benefits for health and weight loss that are superior to low intensity aerobics. You don't have to be able to work out at high intensity for prolonged periods, just in brief sessions. In addition, lower intensity physical activity uses mostly slow-twitch (endurance) muscle fibers. Since fast twitch fibers are also not used much in most activities of daily living, they tend to atrophy at a higher rate as we age. Finally, there is evidence high intensity training is superior for anti-aging and metabolic benefits.

The easiest way to work in some high intensity exercise is doing some stairs briskly during the day. Or you can do Dr. Martin Gibala's short stair climbing workout a couple of times a week, as described in chapter 2. I also mentioned there that you can do some short higher intensity sessions to "get exercise over with" if it is a chore for you. As mentioned in chapter 2, high intensity often happens naturally in sports. But even if it's interval training in a workout it can be enjoyable.

You can do formal interval training, like repeats of 30 seconds fast, with recovery in between. You'll see this in training guides as 8x30, for 8 repetitions of 30 seconds, or 8x30/60 for 8 reps of 30 with 60 seconds rest in between. I like to do mine with a decent amount of recovery, but you can also get a good workout with brief rest. The most famous example is the Tabata workout, developed by exercise scientist Dr Izumi Tabata for the Japanese national speed skating team in the 1990s: 8x20 seconds with 10 seconds easy in between[202]. Dr Tabata's work was a real breakthrough because at the time it was thought that sprint training did not enhance aerobic capacity, but he demonstrated dramatically that it could. If you go hard on the 20 seconds, as you're supposed to, the Tabata protocol gets really challenging towards the 5th rep of so.

I used to enjoy it but had to give it up with my heart issue, it could have triggered afib before my surgery. Now I do more like 8x30/60. My version is sprints on my bike, and I also do an upper body version with heavyhands. A couple of times a week with an easier day the day after works well. An alternative to formal intervals is fartlek (Swedish for "speed-play"), just occasionally picking up the pace for a while when you feel like it. Throw in a power-walk to the next telephone pole when walking, or pick up the pace on uphill sections when hiking.

On Pacing: LISS, But Don't HIIT Or MISS Too Much

Anything done predominantly aerobically is low intensity steady state (LISS). Higher intensity activity exceeds the capacity of the cardiovascular system and the mitochondria in the cells to provide oxygen, so anaerobic glycolysis has to occur: Fuel in the form of muscle glycogen has to be broken without oxygen, a more inefficient process that produces byproducts such as lactate[185]. Moderate intensity steady state (MISS) is continuous activity at a high enough rate that there is significant accumulation of blood lactate. High intensity interval training (HIIT) is intermittent exercise at an anaerobic intensity, with lower intensity recovery in between (as discussed above, for example, the Tabata workout or 8x30). Various authors are coming around to the view that MISS is kind of a no-man's land that is not a good training zone. Spending a lot of time doing MISS is pretty common, though, among serious endurance athletes, and it too much of it can have health drawbacks like a risk of developing Afib. Many examples of this were discussed in <u>The Haywire Heart</u>, by Christopher Case, Dr. John Mandrola, and Lennard Zinn (Chris and Lennard themselves developed Afib). Some in the community of endurance athletes have been in a bit of denial about this issue, so this is an important book.

I also personally find that too much MISS training can feel good while doing it, but can actually leave me kind of wound up so I don't sleep as well at night. This is possibly residual cortisol (a stress hormone) produced in excess by too much volume of fairly intense activity. In contrast, relatively short sessions of HIIT leave me feeling great then relaxed later, while longer sessions of LISS leave me feeling mellow, and both lead to better sleep that night.

Instead of MISS, spending most of your activity at low intensity, and throwing in some high intensity, but avoiding no-man's land is a good approach for good health and fitness (as well as athletic performance). I first learned of this on Clarence Bass's excellent health and fitness website (www.cbass.com). As Clarence put it "I walk and I sprint. I don't do anything in between". This approach has kept Clarence at an elite level of fitness and health for decades, including now at age 80. He does brisk walking in the hills near Albuquerque, not strolls. For high intensity he does intervals on machines like rowers and ski-ergs as well as strength training. He believes in only doing high intensity work less often, like once or at most twice a week, allowing plenty of recovery.

This approach that uses mostly low intensity work and some HIIT, but minimizes MISS, is also called "polarized training". This term was introduced by exercise physiologist Dr. Stephen Seiler[218], who is from Texas but does his work in Norway, a great place to study elite endurance athletes. Polarized training is based on studying the actual training elite endurance athletes do (including runners, rowers, and cross-country skiers), but the effectiveness has also been proven in intervention studies[175].

I think the take away for us non-elites is to go at an easy pace often (during your activities of daily living or scheduled exercise sessions), go hard occasionally (like a couple of times a week, so you have time to recover in between), and don't spend too much time in the no-man's land of MISS in the middle. You can make a big deal out of determining what various training target paces are, using heart rate monitors, or power meters for cycling (they are now starting to be available for running too). But it's easy to just use your breath. As mentioned in the previous chapter, at an easy pace, or LISS, breathing should be comfortable and you should pass the talk test. For high intensity you go hard, and should feel out of breath after each interval, and glad for the recovery period in between.

Legendary coach Bill Bowerman had two other good tips for his runners, both of which are helpful for any activity for the rest of us:
- Easy day/hard day. Always follow a day with a hard workout with an easy day, to allow the body to recover.
- After a hard workout, you should feel "exhilarated not exhausted". A short and sweet interval session is exhilarating for me. If I work out too hard for too long, though, I can feel exhausted.

There are a lot of books out there that claim that HIIT training is superior to LISS, because it gives so much bang for the time buck. This is a valid point, especially if you don't have a LISS activity you particularly enjoy. You can be perfectly healthy getting your low intensity activity from your activities of daily living, and get in great shape quickly just by throwing in some HIIT, maybe twice a week depending on how quickly you recover.

Some authors go so far as to claim LISS is actually harmful, which I don't agree with. It's fine if you like it and don't do too much of it, which could lead to overtraining. I can average more than an hour a day of it without problems. I think the problem is more when people do too much LISS aerobics at the expense of not enough (or any) resistance training and HIIT. The top priority is getting those two done, with LISS optional if you enjoy it.

As a final note on pacing, I recommend going by time, not distance, especially during your longer workouts. I first discovered this when I was biking in Boulder. I despised the wind, and if you live near the front range of the Rockies there is a lot of opportunity to despise it. Then I realized it was because I was always biking a set distance, and if I ended up going against the wind, it was frustrating because it slowed me down. So I switched to going by time. Problem solved. On a windier day I might end up not going as far but because I had gotten my time in I knew it was still a good workout. Andy Burfoot gives reasons for going by time for runners in <u>Run Forever</u>, but his reasoning applies to any endurance activity.

Avoiding Overtraining

For those of us that enjoy exercise (whether cardio, strength, or both), two main training errors are unnecessarily doing too much volume of training, and too much intensity. It's a "more is better" mistake. More can be better, up to a point, but after that you can be breaking your body down too much without giving it enough recovery. Following easy day/hard day is a good start, as is not doing HIIT on too many days. Too high a training volume is another way to overdo. Too much volume or intensity (or both) can lead to overtraining: "Overtraining occurs when a person exceeds their body's ability to recover from strenuous exercise"[186]. It is the recovery that is key. Deana Kastor said that her coach, the legendary Joe Vigil, had a saying "there's no such thing as overtraining, only under-recovery"[207]. There are various signs of overtraining (or under-recovery), including your performance getting worse, increased resting heart rate in the morning, persistent muscle soreness, susceptibility to illness, and grumpiness. It's time to dial the training back when any of this happens. This is more of an issue for pretty serious athletes.

Challenge Yourself (But Choose Your Challenge Wisely)

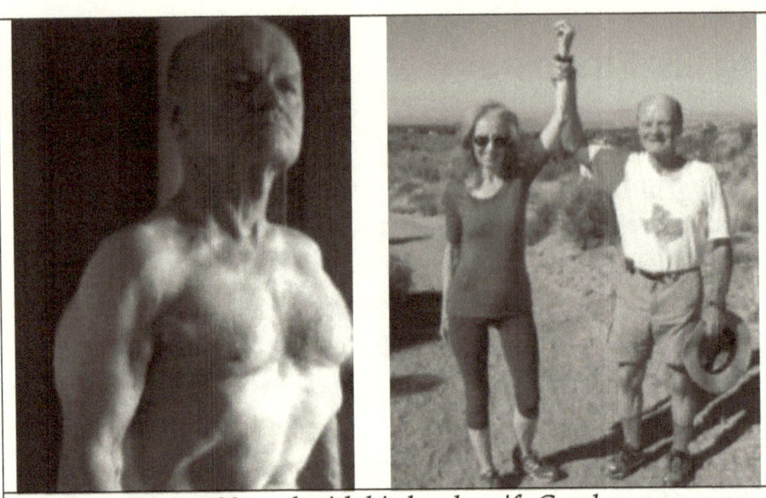

Clarence Bass at 80, and with his lovely wife Carol (www.cbass.com

I got this idea from Clarence Bass, in his book <u>Challenge Yourself</u>. It can be much easier to motivate yourself to be physically active if there is some challenge you're pointing towards. But we can tend to have a "bigger is better" mentality and choose tests like marathons, century rides, or climbing Mt. Whitney. These can be good "bucket list" items. I'm glad I did one marathon. Not so sure about three. The problem with doing a lot of these is that in trying to build up to a big goal, you can cross the line into "chronic cardio", or high volume training (often at MISS pace). This can get you very fit but not necessarily healthier.

It's better to have a goal that motivates you to do more optimal training that supports good health. When I first read how Clarence uses a two minute session on the Concept2 rower as his challenge, I tried the bicycling equivalent: trying to get faster climbing some short but steep hills in my town, and comparing my result with my age group on www.strava.com.

This was a humbling experience, there are a lot of fit people in my area. One of the local "king of the mountain" titles belongs to the great mountain biker Ned Overend who is in my age group, so I'm obviously never going to get close to that. But it still challenges me to do better and motivates me when I'm doing my bike intervals. When Clarence read this section he commented "Key is to remember that the only competitor that counts is YOU". Thanks for the reminder, Clarence. The idea is to motivate us to keep striving, not compare ourselves to others.

Lots of people thrive on longer challenges, including marathons, ultramarathons, and long triathlons. I'm not trying to discourage anyone from that, but for many of us excitement, fun, and good health can come from shorter events. Julie Carter, a British champion fellrunner, discusses the philosophy of inspiring ourselves with challenges in her inspiring book <u>Running The Red Line</u>. In her opinion, which I share, the key is to explore beyond your current comfort zone. This can be by going longer that you're comfortable with or harder. I do sometimes like to push myself longer than I'm used to, for example on hikes. This can earn you superb views in places you've never seen before. But more often I'm going harder than currently comfortable in shorter challenges. These are not mutually exclusive and you can pursue both without overtraining. For example, once a week go longer at a brisk but comfortable pace, and one or two other times go harder for shorter.

Stretching

Slow static stretches are relaxing and help keep you limber as you age. I think it is best to learn these from a qualified instructor like a yoga or pilates teacher that can correct your form. When you've learned a simple series of them you can do them at home. There are also good beginner instructional videos for stretching, and yoga classes at gyms and adult ed centers.

Static stretching is not the only way to stay flexible. Clarence Bass describes his morning routine which takes all important joints through their ranges of motion (www.cbass.com/getupandmove.htm). Suzanne Wylde's book <u>Moving Stretch: Work Your Fascia to Free Your Body</u> describes an alternate approach where you more your body through various positions with muscles lightly resisting each other. Muscles that are stretched while tense are in eccentric contraction, which provides a good stretch for their surrounding connective tissues (fascia). There are also some introductory videos of her approach on her website: www.movingstretch.com.

Resistance training exercises with full range of motion (like a full squat) provide flexibility as well. I read somewhere that the flexibility of all athletes on the US summer Olympic team was once tested. Gymnasts, not surprisingly, were the most flexible. But the weight lifters came in second. So much for the stereotype of weight lifters being "musclebound"!

Balance

A neglected aspect of fitness that becomes more important with aging is balance. This is another area where decline occurs with age, and makes older people more likely to fall. Young people can stand on one foot with their eyes closed easily for a minute. I can do it for about 10 seconds. I knew my balance had gotten worse, but it was driven home to me recently on a hike. Our group came to the informal bridge shown. There were two logs about 4 inches in diameter, one slightly lower than the other, but otherwise stable. In crossing this I was one of the worst in the group, which included people a few years older than me.

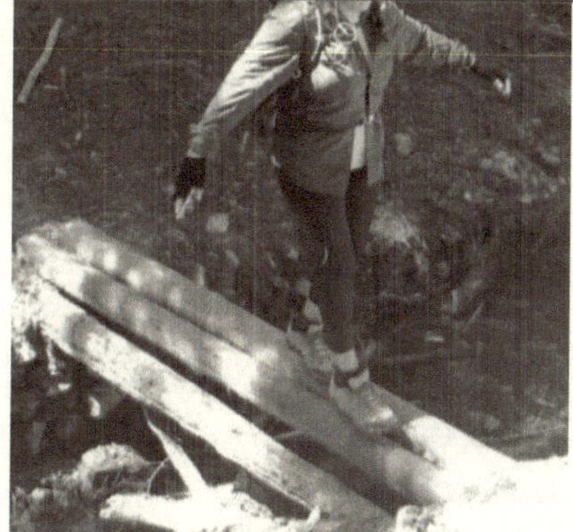

A balance challenge (informal bridge over Fall Creek, Henry Cowell Redwoods State Park, Felton, Ca).

Balance probably declines worse than other physical capacities with age, maybe because it is a downward spiral. As it degrades, we unconsciously get more timid about challenging it. Fortunately, as I read in Jim Klopman's book Balance is Power[196], it responds quickly to training. Jim has some brain symptoms from concussions he suffered from falls in thrill sports in his youth decades ago. He improved his own symptoms dramatically with advanced balance training, and consulted with brain health expert Dr. Daniel Amen, author of many self-help books on the brain including The Brain Warrior's Way.

Dr. Amen feels that balance training is an important tool for using neuro-plasticity (the ability of the brain to make new connections, no matter how old we are) to heal the brain. Balance is Power has 3 levels of training, and it only took me a couple of days to get a lot better at level I and proceed into level II. With continued progress this has spilled over into my hiking, mountain biking, and other activities.

One activity that I recommend adding to Jim's suggestions is the walking lunge. This is a good way to build leg strength but also requires good balance. Watching contestants at the recent Crossfit games making lunges look easy while holding heavy kettlebells overhead inspired me to try it. As expected I found it to be a good test (even without weights) from a strength standpoint, but also surprisingly challenging for balance.

Tips on Some Specific Activities

Running

Most people do not feel comfortable running for extended periods right away. The run-walk technique is a way to get through that. Say you can run for a minute now without getting too much out of breath and would like to build up to 30 minutes continuously. You could walk for a few minutes to warm up, then alternate a few intervals of 1 minute running followed by 1 minute walking, then do a cooldown walk. This might progress like this over several weeks:

- 5 min warmup, 5x(1 minute run then 1 minute walk), then 5 minute cooldown = 20 minutes
- Week 2 repeat the run-walk 6x = 22 minutes total
- Week 3 repeat the run-walk 7x = 24 minutes total
- Week 4 repeat the run-walk 8x = 26 minutes total
- Week 5 repeat the run-walk 9x = 28 minutes total
- Week 6 repeat the run-walk 10x = 30 minutes total

Now you could keep it at 10 but start shortening your walks and lengthening your runs, like 1:15 run, 45 sec walk, etc., until you phase out the walk breaks and end up with 5 min warmup, 20 minute run, and then 5 minute cooldown. Then you can start replacing part of your warmup and cooldown with slower running, until the workout becomes a 30 minute run. At that point, hopefully you are enjoying running, and could continue to improve either by making it longer or going faster.

For a lot of tips and inspiration on getting started on running plus making it last a lifetime, I highly recommend Andy Burfoot's <u>Run Forever</u>. Andy won the Boston Marathon in 1968, and, even more relevant to our topic of aging gracefully, just returned at 71 to run it again on the 50th anniversary of his victory. The simple run-walk plan above is what worked for me when I started out. Andy has a different plan which also looks good and I'd recommend it especially if it's hard for you to run for 1 minute straight at the beginning. Even though he feels running in the hills can be a good workout and more enjoyable, especially if you can get out on trails, Andy recommends that beginners stick to the flat at least until you are used to running for 30 minutes straight. You can still get good scenery in parks.

And don't forget about run-walk in the long term. Olympian and coach Jeff Galloway has been suggesting it for many years as a way to get through longer running events more pleasantly and with less recovery needed after, but you still get a great workout (see, for example, his book <u>Run Walk Run Method</u>). For example you can take a short walk break every mile while running a marathon. I never tried it, because I thought running a marathon "didn't count" unless I ran the whole way (a variation on Dr. Segars's psychological "doesn't count" trap, discussed in chapter 2). I wish I had, maybe I wouldn't have been so sore for weeks after the marathon if I had. Andy Burfoot is also an enthusiast advocate of long-term use of the run-walk method.

Heavyhands

This is a way to get a bit more of a workout from your walk, as well as some upper-body exercise. It can also make it more fun if you like the feel of it, as I do. Heavyhands was invented by Dr. Leonard Schwartz[138]. He was in his 50s, overweight, and trying to get back into shape. He didn't like running and didn't feel he could get enough intensity walking. Since cross country skiers have some of the best aerobic capacity of any elite athletes, he figured the four limbed motion was the key, so tried adding hand weights to his walking. He also came up with a lot of variations to get more muscles involved, and named the activity heavyhands. He did this exclusively as his exercise, and got extremely fit (and buff) and stayed that way until his death from lymphoma at age 84 in 2010. We lost a great man with his passing, and unfortunately his body of work on exercise is no longer as well-known as it deserves to be.

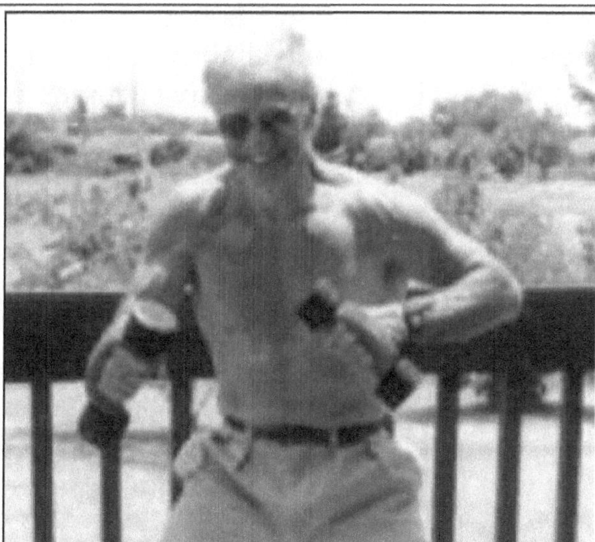

Dr. Leonard Schwartz, inventor of HeavyHands
(www.cbass.com/LeonardSchwartz.htm)

I do heavier training with bands (or at the gym) for some of the key muscle groups as discussed above, and also do heavyhands. Based on Dr. Schwartz's example, heavyhands is probably enough by itself if you don't like conventional strength training. Brisk walking with a normal gait, swinging arm weights, is a great workout. It's essentially your normal arm movement in a controlled manner while walking briskly, but with weights in your hands. Dr. Schwartz preferred saying "pumping" to "swinging" to imply a more controlled motion.

Depending on how uninhibited you are in public, you can also do a more vigorous arm motion: a normal arm swing comes up to about your waist. Adding more vertical motion, like up to the level of your chest or shoulders, is more challenging. I also add a punch motion (when no one is looking) that gets in a trunk twist and is a good way to build stamina for kayaking.

Another fun one is mimicking the motion of skate-style cross country skiing: step forward and slightly diagonally to the left with your left foot while simultaneously swinging both weights up to the front (the higher you go, the better the workout, I go about head high). Then step off and slightly diagonally to the right with your right foot while simultaneously swinging both weights down and back. After doing this for a few strides, switch sides and move the weights up with the right foot and down with the left. The arm movement is similar to the poling action in skate-style skiing.

You can also get a good combination quad, ab, back, shoulder, and arm workout with double-poling, which can be done stationary. Start upright, raise the arms forward to at least head height. Then crouch down as you swing the weights vigorously back. Then stand upright and swing the weights vigorously to head height. This gets more of a workout for the front shoulder muscles and biceps because they are fighting gravity more. You can balance this out by doing the same motion but using resistance bands mounted to an eyebolt high in the wall. As you crouch down and swings the arms back, you are pull the bands vigorously down and back. As you stand back up and swing the arms up, the bands are giving you some assistance. So this uses more of the abs, triceps, lats, and rear shoulder muscles. This is an inexpensive alternative to Concept2's excellent ski erg machine (which I now have access to at the gym- I love the smooth action and long range of motion). If you want inspiration for this exercise, you can find videos on the web of cross country skiers double-poling in a sprint finish, or on the ski erg.

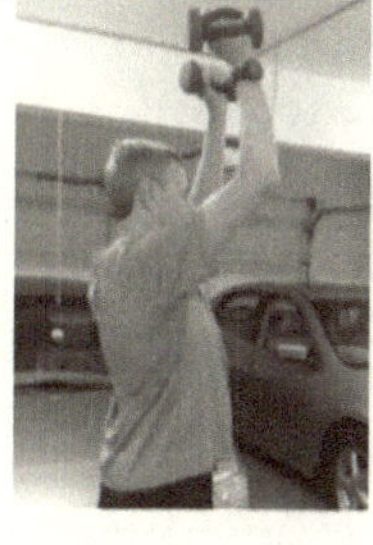	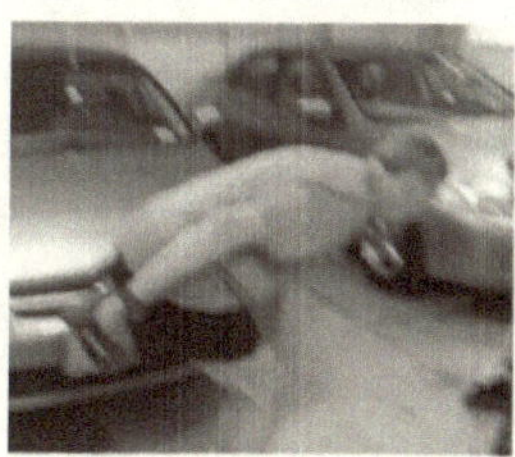	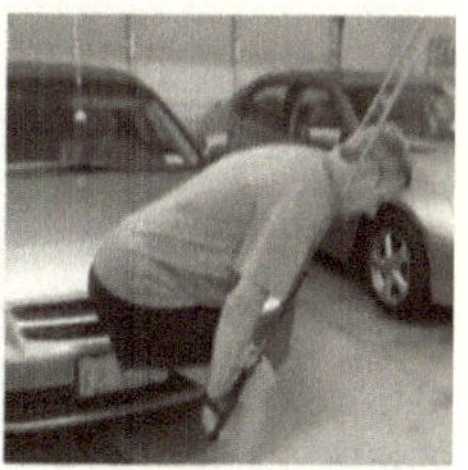
Vigorously swing weights up while straightening torso	Vigorously swing weights down and back while bending torso and crouching	Alternative with resistance bands
Double Ski Poling Exercise		

There are many other exercises in Dr. Schwartz's book Heavyhands Walking (which you can still find on Amazon). If you are embarrassed doing some of the other motions in public, you could stick to walking outdoors with the weights without too high of an arm swing, which looks perfectly natural, and do alternative movements in the privacy of your home.

You can also do interval training with hand weights, just do the walking with arm swing, for example, but faster and/or with somewhat heavier weights. Alternate going at a more leisurely pace with doing the motion quite vigorously for around 30 seconds. Start out with small weights that don't interfere with your arm swing, as little as 1 lb. If you do enjoy it, over time you'll get a bit stronger and can increase the weights. I "cruise" with 3 or 4 lbs. now, and use 6 lbs. for intervals.

I suggest weights with straps that are readily available in sizes up to 5 lbs., because this spares your grip and prevents cramping. Dr. Schwartz invented Heavyhands weights specifically for this purpose that are adjustable in weight; millions of these were sold by AMF in the 1980s. They are hard to find nowadays, but some are still available on ebay. Another option is that there are companies making weights with straps including GetFit, Gymenist, Spri, Tone Fitness, WalkPlus, and Weider. You can find weights in sizes 1 through 5 lbs by searching for "walking dumbbells" or "walking weights". There is also an easy way to make your own wrist straps described in the figure.

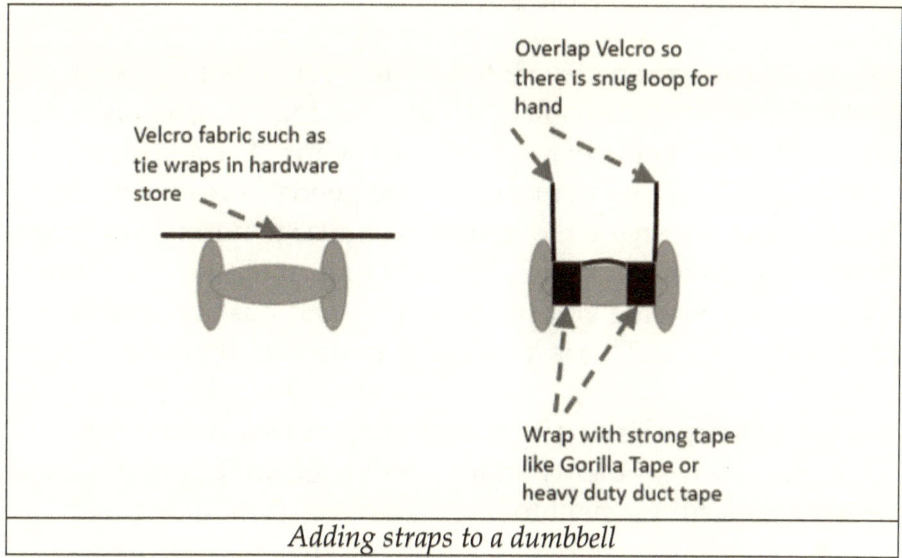

Adding straps to a dumbbell

If you have given Heavyhands a try with one of these options and like it, you may want to treat yourself to the cadillac version of hand weights offered by Michael Senoff on his website www.weightedhands.com. His are adjustable in weight, comfortable and very nicely made, with ergonomic grips and custom fitted straps. Michael's website is also a treasure trove of information about heavyhands and Dr. Schwartz, including interviews with people who knew him well. You can get as vigorous as you'd like with a heavyhands workout. If I were to walk briskly down the street with 6 pound weights or so swinging up to my chest or higher, I'd get tired in a few minutes, but I could work up to doing it longer if desired. Or I can do a less vigorous arm swing, and throw in high intensity intervals with faster walking and higher arm swing.

Walking with Poles (Nordic Walking)

Another way to add some intensity to your walking is with poles, sometimes also called Nordic walking because it is similar to the motion of cross country skiing. The adjustable walking poles found at most sporting goods stores are fine for starting out. The basic movement is similar to normal walking with a vigorous arm swing, but as your arm reaches the limit of its forward swing you plant the pole and push on it as your arm swings back. This is a lot easier to do than describe!

There is plenty of instruction, including videos, online, for example at www.americannordicwalking.com/technique. I use this as a supplement to heavyhands. Basic walking with hand weights uses more of the front shoulders, chest, and biceps muscles because they are working against gravity while raising the weight.

Pole walking uses more of the complementary muscles (rear shoulders, lats, and triceps) as you are pushing back on the pole. You can make this movement pretty high intensity by walking briskly and pushing back hard, or by doing it uphill.

Biking

I recommend a more upright bike like a "comfort bike" or a hybrid for most people, especially starting out. These have flat bar handlebars that feel more natural than road-bike style "drop bars". If you don't think you'll ever want to go off pavement, a "flat bar road bike" is a good choice, because they have skinnier tires and you can go pretty fast. Otherwise a hybrid with fatter tires and at least front suspension will do well on road or dirt.

An interesting option if you are not used to biking is a bike with cranks a little further forward like cruisers or the Electra Townie (which is similar to the classic position on Dutch bikes). You can put your feet flat on the ground without getting off the saddle. I also think they look cool. My mom never rode a bike much as a kid and tried to take up biking as an adult. On her first ride she fell at the first stop sign because she didn't remember she had to get off the saddle for her feet to reach the ground. She scraped her knee pretty badly and was turned off to cycling for life. This would not have happened on the Townie!

Other manufacturers have come out with bikes with this position now too. Electra has also paid homage to Dutch bikes with the "Amsterdam", similar to the Townie but with fenders, a rack, and a full chain guard and a skirt guard. In Holland and other countries like Denmark where lots of cycling is done for utility purposes, this is the typical type of bike. I love the Dutch name for them: Omafiets ("Grandma's bike). People cycle in their everyday clothes, including dresses, not special cycling clothes. This is nicely described in <u>Building the Cycling City: The Dutch Blueprint for Urban Vitality</u> by Melissa and Chris Bruntlett.

There is an interesting and fun comparison of flat bar vs. drop bar road bikes by the guys at global cycling network on youtube (www.youtube.com/watch?v=Q6-yz1qJrUc) entitled "Flat Bar Vs Drop Bar Road Bikes | Comfort, Speed & Ease". I loved their high-tech tests. They concluded drop bars get the nod on speed while flat bars are a bit better on agility, like riding in traffic.

I have a couple of things to add from my experience. It is true drop bars offer multiple riding positions ("the tops", "the hoods", and "the drops"). And todays bikes with drop bars have a lot of padding on the brake hoods, making that a comfortable position. Flat bars have only one position, but you can add another with bar ends.

Many of the people I ride with have drop bars, but I almost never see them riding in the drops, so they don't use the speed advantage. You can also get a speed boost by putting aerobar clip-ons on your flat bars, which is what I do for time trialing. This is a good idea if you do a combination of city and country riding. The flat bars are great to make you nimble around traffic, while the aerobars let you cruise fast in the country. That worked well for me when I had a bike commute that started in the country and ended downtown.

There is only one thing I miss from drop bars: going fast downhill. You definitely don't want to be in the aerobars on steep downhills because you don't have enough control- it feels squirrely. In the drops you can be aero, with your fingers near the brakes if needed, and with great control. The closest you can get to that with flat bars is bending your arms so you can hunch over the bars, which I find uncomfortable after a while. All of this is less of an issue for me in my later years because I'm not as intrepid of a descender as I once was. While this advice, and the demonstrations on the youtube video, may be helpful, everyone is different when it comes to comfort. If you are just starting out and are unsure of flat bars vs drop, I recommend finding out for yourself with a long test ride of both.

Saddle comfort is a big issue. You can start out with shorter rides and gradually increase them, as your butt toughens up over time. Don't worry, that happens internally, it's not like you get giant visible callouses on your butt. Well-designed modern saddles address an important issue of pressure in the genital area for both men and women.

Your weight should be transferred to the saddle mainly from the "sit bones" (ischial tuberosity) and not by the soft tissue in the genital region. And pressure on the perineal nerve should be minimum. Solutions include cutouts and ridges under the sit bones with pressure relieving trough in between. A saddle which puts pressure on the perineal nerve can cause temporary penile numbness in men and possible longer term effects. Pressure in the genital area can cause vaginal discomfort in women. A good saddle should prevent all of the above and your bike shop should help you with fitting one.

Another comfort option I enjoy is standing up to pedal. The easiest thing to do is just standing up occasionally for a short period to take a "butt break". Or, if you have big enough gears, like a 48 tooth chainring up front and an 11 tooth gear in the back, you can pedal standing for longer periods at a comfortable pace. With flat bars you can also make the position nice and upright with bar ends. I just gang two pairs together as shown in the picture below, so when I stand up I'm not hunched over. There is zero discomfort pedaling this way, and I find the motion as relaxing as running. It's a good workout too.

The longest I've stood for is about 2½ hours. I decided that since this felt kind of like running, I'd see how long it took me to standup-pedal for 26.2 miles, and it took 2 hours 28 minutes. And I felt great afterwards because there was no pounding. So now I can brag I'm a 2:28 marathoner (ok, maybe with a little asterisk next to it).

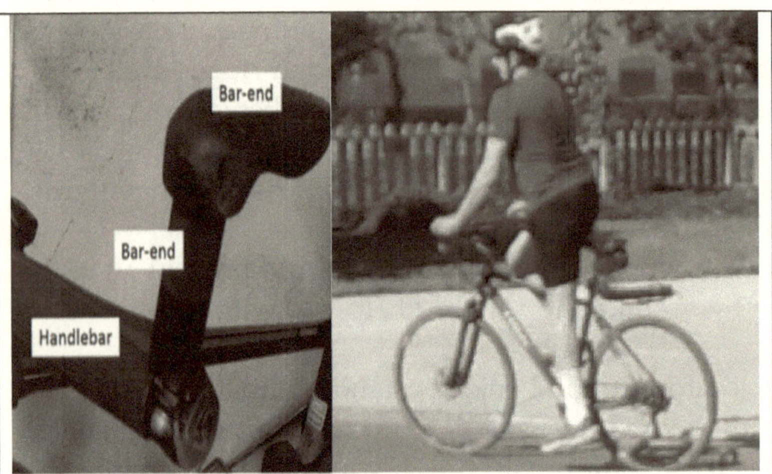

Handlebar extender for standing up to pedal. The first bar end has a straight shaft with the same diameter as a handle bar. The second (upper) bar end then clamps to it. When standing, you are comfortably upright while holding the upper bar end

Another option for comfort is riding a recumbent, with the downside that they are pricier than upright bikes since it's a smaller market. It's important to find a good dealer and go on long test rides. For a while I had back and neck issues on conventional bikes, compounded by the fact I spent too much time hunched over a computer with poor posture, and recumbents worked well to solve this. I had good luck with Rans and Bacchetta recumbents, but there are a lot of good brands reviewed at www.bentrideronline.com.

One warning is that a recumbent is not a guarantee of comfort. There is a phenomenon called "recumbutt" because you are sitting on your glute muscles, which can interfere with the blood flow to them while they are working. This can lead to restricted blood flow to the muscles (ischemia), which causes an achy feeling. I had this badly with a couple of brands, which is why long test rides are a good idea. I was fine on the Rans and Bacchetta bikes, but everyone's anatomy is a bit different.

Some people who are older have balance issues on bikes, and a trike is a good alternative. This does not have to be one of those big upright ones with the basket between the rear wheels. There are also higher performance recumbent trikes, some of which also fold for transport (www.bentrideronline.com).

One last thing on the subject of bikes is electric-assist, for which there are many quality options available now. It needs a full book to do this topic justice, and you need a recently written one because the technology is evolving quickly. <u>Ebikes: A Buyer's Guide: Understand Ebikes And Buy The One That's Best For You</u>, by Paul Fox is a good concise recent book. Electric assist bikes still let you get a good workout, they just help you to go faster or climb hills better.

I have a friend who is now 80 that has one, he describes it as "always having a tailwind". When he was 65 and I was 50 he could leave me in the dust on a bike, especially climbing. Now he's slowing down a bit so has trouble keeping up on group rides. Electric assist solved the problem.

Another good use regardless of your age is commuting. You can use a high level of assist on your way to work and show up fast without sweating on your way there. On your way home you can get a good workout by using less assist. Finally, they are useful in extending your range. I do lots of errands in Morgan Hill on my bike because it is a pretty compact town. Sometimes I need to get to further away locations that would take too long by bike, but electric assist would increase my average speed and make it more feasible to get there.

Chapter 4-My Take on Diet

I became mildly interested in a healthy eating in my early adulthood and have been reading up on it ever since. In trying to figure things out for myself, I have read extensively on various diets, with an open mind. I do not take what any of the authors say at face value but always try to chase down the underlying science. In this chapter I go over what I have learned and what works for me.

My Eating Story

My own odyssey to find a healthier diet began in earnest when I was about 45, back in the late 1990s, when "middle aged spread" started to accumulate, even though I was very active physically. I was able to get down to my desired weight if I was diligent about exercising and watching my calorie intake, but always had to fight off cravings, especially my sweet tooth.

This went on for many years until around the end of 2016 when I had a physical, and my blood work wasn't great. Bad cholesterol too high, good cholesterol too low, and triglycerides too high. My doc was especially concerned about my triglycerides, and told me to cut back on carbs. That led me to intensify my search for a healthy and sustainable way of eating.

But let's start at the beginning. Grandma did most of the cooking as Mom was the breadwinner. We followed what was a typical American diet at the time. But there was nowhere near as much fast food available back then. A McDonald's came in a few miles away when I was about 8, but we considered going there a special treat, maybe once a month. At McD's back then you could get a small hamburger, small fries, and soda or a milkshake. No big macs yet. And they used to brag about how many millions of hamburgers had been sold, not billions.

We didn't go out to eat that often in general because of the expense, and because Grandma loved to cook. It was mostly meat and taters; vegetables might be a can of cream style corn or peas. The exception was in the summer when Jersey's local produce was available and it earned its nickname "the garden state": amazing local beefsteak tomatoes and corn on the cob headed the list. We also ate a decent amount of fruit.

We drank very little soda because my grandma made a version of iced tea that tasted like the "black tea lemonade" they serve at Starbucks (only she didn't charge 4 dollars a glass for hers). This probably didn't save us too much in the sugar department compared to soda, though, because I remember her dumping sugar into the pitcher by the scoopful when she made it

I do remember having a coke from time to time, in its 6 ½ oz. bottle. If you really wanted to splurge you got a large size soda, which was 12 oz. back then. Refined food was definitely creeping in but grandma mostly cooked from scratch. She made a lot of pies, with the crust made with lard, until that amazing invention Crisco came out in 1960. I remember her ladling that glop from the big red can. There were early TV dinners like Swanson turkey in its little aluminum tray with compartments, but again that was only an occasional special treat. No junk food or soda machines in the schools. I took a bag lunch to school, a sandwich on wonder bread, an apple, and some of Grandma's cookies.

I was 18 and in college when Frances Moore Lappé's book Diet for a Small Planet came out, arguing that eating plants is more efficient than meat as far as resource consumption, appealing reasoning to a budding engineer. So I decided to be a vegetarian, despite the fact I had no idea how to cook nor knew anything about nutrition other than what I learned from that one book.

There were no tofu, veggie burgers or other meat alternatives in the supermarket back then, and you couldn't ask for the vegan option at a restaurant, they wouldn't have known what you were talking about. While I hung in there for about 2 years as a vegetarian, I survived mostly on cheese pizza and meatless Italian dishes like manicotti, which fortunately are plentiful and superb in New Jersey.

After I graduated, Karen and I moved to Pennsylvania. I gave my vegetarianism up, so it was back to the standard American diet. Only now fast food was readily available, and I partook of plenty of it. I was pretty active in running and bicycling by this time, so I was able to keep this up for many years without gaining weight. I'd go for a half hour run at lunch and I could eat whatever I wanted.

I would visit my brother Bill in Phoenix and we'd go out for a brisk morning run, burning a few hundred calories maybe, then go to a nice restaurant and proceed to inhale a few thousand calories for breakfast. When you're active and young that math somehow works out. It stopped working after I was about 45. The pounds gradually crept on until I was 25 pounds overweight.

Karen and I both decided to fight the onset of middle aged spread by joining Weight Watchers.
They have a point system which back then consisted of tracking the calories, fat, and fiber of your food, and that would get converted to points by a little cardboard slipstick calculator they gave you. You were allocated an amount of points for the day based on your current weight. Remember, I'm an engineer, so I treated this as an optimization problem. What's the maximum I can stuff into my face without exceeding my points budget?

It turned out the answer, based on the formula WW used back then, was to go very low fat. So I ended up close to following the Pritikin diet, which was well known at the time, because Nathan Pritikin had good success with heart disease patients on this diet[107]. It did not, however, have a particularly good rep for flavor. The movie "Sister Act" with Whoopi Goldberg came out in 1992, where she is on the run from the mob, hiding out in a convent pretending to be a nun. When she tastes her first spoonful of food in the convent she makes a face and says "what is this, a Pritikin order"?

This was in the middle of the low-fat era. I read up on nutrition at this time and there was plenty of logic behind this approach if done properly. You were supposed to eat lots of fruits, veggies, legumes, and minimally processed grains, and eat less meat and leaner cuts of it, and avoid processed food and junk like soda or cookies. Pritikin and others like Dean Ornish never said it was ok to eat sugary foods (like "snackwell" cookies) just because it's low fat.

Unfortunately, that was not how low-fat was interpreted by the mainstream and the results had a disastrous effect on the nation's waistline. In the early 2000's the pendulum swung from low-fat to low-carb, but then the food industry jumped on that too, offering low-carb ice cream and carbwell cookies instead of low-fat ice cream and snackwell cookies. Low-carb junk didn't work out any better than low-fat junk, so the relentless progress of the collective waistline continued unabated.

My Pritikin-like diet worked great for me. I was able to lose all the weight and keep it off for several years, as long as I exercised a lot and diligently counted my Weight Watchers points. Then it gradually crept back on as I again became less careful about what ate. I fought it for many years, keeping my weight and waistline reasonable close to what I wanted (as long as I exercised enough) but always with a few more pounds around the waist than I would have liked. The problem was that I still had cravings, enough to get me to eat too many snacks at night if I wasn't careful, and need Tums at bedtime.

Let me go into a little more of what I mean by cravings. I have a sweet tooth and a tendency towards binge eating. Not super bad binges, but enough to get me to eat several snacks after dinner and need the aforementioned Tums, as well as torpedo any weight loss efforts. I'd sit down in my nice comfy chair to watch a good show or sporting event.

Then the little voice would start in- I call it my gremlin. "How about some ice cream. Just a little bit. Oh c'mon, it's low fat what could it hurt?" I'd fight that off for a few minutes then go all right, damn it, I'll eat a small amount of ice cream. Back to the chair, eat the ice cream. A few minutes later "how about some cookies? Oh c'mon you've already blown your calorie budget for the day, you may as well go for it". Sly little bugger, that gremlin. Some nights I'd fight it off completely, sometimes it would win multiple times and I'd end up with the tums or pepto bismol.

But whether or not it won, this constant battle was a pain in the ass! If I could gut it out and go for a stretch of a few weeks of winning the battle, I could lose some weight, but the gremlin would be back with a vengeance and I'd backslide. But I could still keep things in check as long as I exercised a lot. This went on until the physical and the bad blood work in 2016 that I mentioned above.

OK, Doc says eat less carbs. Reading on nutrition had been a hobby all this time so I tried the carb restriction approach recommended in Dr. Grant Schofield's book <u>What the Fat</u>[136], which also recommended lots of veggies and cutting out all junk. I followed this for a couple of weeks and felt great, noticing right away that I had no cravings, so eating this way was effortless and sustainable, and I readily kept it up for 3 weeks. So far so good!

But it didn't stop there, because there was the complication of my aortic stenosis that I talked about in chapter 1. I was motivated to see if there was anything I could do with diet to reverse it or slow its progression, so I did some research on that. The chance turns out to be rather slim based on current knowledge, but there was some anecdotal evidence that following Dr. Caldwell Esselstyn's heart disease reversal diet might help[203]. This is a whole food plant based (wfpb) diet which also emphasizes very low fat. I decided to give that a try.

I discussed the palatability reputations of the Pritikin and Ornish diets above and this one could have the same issues if you were strict enough with it. You are supposed to sauté in vegetable broth so you don't use any added oil for cooking. Dr. Esselstyn's wife is a great cook so there are many good recipes in the book. And his son, Rip Esselstyn, wrote a book <u>The Engine 2 Diet</u>. Rip was a firefighter serving with Engine 2 in Austin, Texas, and got his engine-mates to eat wfpb, improving all their cholesterol and triglyceride numbers considerably in the process. There are a lot of good recipes in this book also, and between the two books it is entirely possible you could eat this way enjoyably.

I'm not a good cook so I gave up after a couple of botched attempts. I then cheated a little on the oil, using a refillable sprayer so I could use a reduced amount of oil for stirfrys, and allowing some oil in salad dressings, so I did not meet Dr. Esselstyn's very strict 10% fat target, but was probably reasonably close. This allowed me to come up with more palatable food choices that were easy for a mediocre cook like me to make.

Needless to say, switching to this diet was a major flip from one end of the spectrum to the other, essentially "restrict your carbs, but plenty of fat is ok" to "eat all the carbs you want as long as they're all from whole foods, but watch the fat". I felt great on it also. I still had no cravings, so it was also effortless to sustain. What was in common between this and the low carb diet was emphasizing whole foods and minimizing processed foods. I didn't go from eating quarter pounders with cheese, but leave off the bun, to eating veggie burgers but the bun is ok. I went from salads and stirfrys with lots of veggies that had meat in them, to salads and stirfrys with lots of veggies and with plant-based protein sources like beans and tofu.

I continued on this diet for several months, gradually losing 15 pounds in the process, and when I went to my Doc for a follow-up, my bloodwork was superb, including good triglycerides. One important thing to point out is that I didn't start to lose weight eating this way until after a few weeks. But since my major objective was transitioning to a healthy diet, not weight loss, I was able to avoid being discouraged by that. Gradual weight loss did kick in after that. Unfortunately none of this helped the heart valve, which progressed to the point of needing the aforementioned surgery in August 2017.

But I decided my way of eating "ain't broke, don't fix it" so stayed with it. I had another reason to continue to be strict about diet: as I mentioned in chapter 1, I got a "tissue" (bovine) replacement valve, and tissue valves eventually get calcified and no longer open property, just like the original valve they replaced. The mechanism is unclear but thought to be similar to how calcified coronary plaque forms, so a "heart healthy" diet may well also be a "heart valve replacement healthy diet", and allow me to get more years out of the replacement.

But I'd also had an angiogram prior to surgery that showed my coronary arteries were clear, so I did relax about fat as long as it's "good fat". Dean Ornish points out in his book <u>The Spectrum</u> that while very low fat has been shown to work for reversal of coronary artery blockages, it's not needed for those of us just trying to stay healthy.

One thing that puzzled me was what had happened to the cravings. I had thought they were just something psychological that you'd have to fight off with discipline and good habits. From my description of my "gremlin" above, it sounds pretty psychological to me. It would have been tempting to think "maybe a shrink can put me on some meds, or a support group or meditation might help". But the little gremlin went away completely when I fixed my diet.

Then I read Dr. David Ludwig's book <u>Always Hungry?</u>, which explains the biological source of cravings and presents an eating approach to eliminate them. The first step is a stricter diet to address the cravings, and then you can see what works for you long term. It turns out the restricted-carb diet I'd followed prior to doing wfpb was pretty similar to Dr. Ludwig's first step, while wfpb qualifies for his longer term approach to preventing cravings, as long as you minimize eating refined carbs.

So I'd blundered into the equivalent of his approach on my own. But I now knew I need to be diligent about the "whole foods" part, especially avoiding refined carbs. Shunning these makes me to able to enjoy eating without having to battle cravings.

What I eat now

I follow a mostly wfpb diet, and I am very strict about the whole foods, especially avoiding refined carbs. When I "stray" it is to allow some oils (like extra virgin olive oil or expeller-pressed canola oil), and some animal foods. I do use healthier varieties of meat substitutes like tofurky (which is just organic tofu, spices, and some healthy oil) but try to avoid more highly processed versions such as those containing soy protein isolate.

I eat a lot of stirfrys, salads, and soups as my main course. I eat whole grain cereals (or pseudo-grains like buckwheat), cooked grains like brown and wild rice, Trader Joe's sprouted whole grain breads, and nuts and seeds (mostly raw). I eat a lot of fruit, some of it dry (unsweetened). With both nuts, seeds, and dry fruits it's easy to go overboard with the calories, and to avoid this I carefully watch the quantities.

Creamy sauces can be made without oil using avocado, almond yogurt, almond milk or cashews. I eat a decent amount of fat, maybe about 30% of my calories. As discussed below, wfpb can be tuned lower fat by adding in more starchy foods (still unrefined) and cutting back on fat sources, or higher fat by cutting back on starch. I personally find that if I go too low on fat, cravings can return.

I don't eat dairy except occasionally in coffee, and I eat a lot less meat and other animal foods than the average American.

I have several reasons for this. First, there are some long term health and longevity concerns with excess consumption of animal foods discussed in the appendix.

Also Americans are eating 1.5 times the amount of meat and more than 7 times the amount of cheese compared to a hundred years ago[173] (a time when the population was much leaner than now) so it seems sensible to cut back. Finally, although the evidence for the connection between saturated fat and heart disease may be murkier than previously thought (also discussed in the appendix), there is still evidence of a connection between saturated fat and calcification of heart valves, and I would like my replacement valve to last as long as possible.

This is what works for me. But I also firmly believe diet is not one size fits all. For example there are some people that are intolerant to legumes or grains. Alternatives like the paleo diet may work better for them, as described in Rob Wolf's book <u>Wired to Eat</u>[81]. But that diet is flexible as well, as Rob describes, and does not necessarily need to be higher in meat consumption. Because both are adjustable, there can actually be considerable overlap between wfpb and paleo. And both emphasize whole foods and minimizing processed foods. I'll go over alternatives to wfpb below.

Overview of Healthy Eating Suggestions

I use "diet" and "way of eating" interchangeably. I do not believe in short term fixes like "I'm going on a diet", I'm referring to permanent lifestyle change. I delve into the details of what I have learned below.

But here's a simpler overview. There is a lot of hype, misinformation, and conflicting information on nutrition in the media, and government guidelines change over time and often can be influenced by the food industry more than based on real science. And even authors who try to base their results on sound science don't agree on everything.

This causes so much bewilderment that lots of people throw up their hands and keep eating the Standard American Diet (which has the appropriate acronym SAD) or its equivalent in other countries. And that's not working out so well for us, with a large percentage of the population overweight or obese and associated medical issues like metabolic syndrome, heart disease, and type II diabetes.

My approach is in 3 steps:
- Stick to some simple rules for healthy eating.
- Go through a temporary eating program I call the "reset", designed to fix any metabolic dysfunction caused by years of eating the SAD, so that food cravings are eliminated. This also allows you to fine tune your diet to what works best for you. You may not lose much (or any) weight during this period, and have to be ok with that. The primary goal is to fix your metabolism and get rid of cravings. Gradual and sustained weight loss will kick in as a byproduct of that. I also present an alternative to more gradually change your way of eating if the reset seems too drastic.
- Continue on with healthy eating until you reach your desired weight, and then maintain at that weight with ease.

None of this will result in rapid weight loss. Instead, cravings will be addressed from the outset, so it will be easier and more enjoyable to follow a long-term healthy way of eating. This will lead to gradual weight loss if needed, and then successful maintenance of your ideal weight. But as explained in Dr. David Ludwig's book <u>Always Hungry?</u>, would you like to quickly lose weight in a month, then spend the next 11 months struggling to maintain it while fighting cravings, or would you rather gradually lose the weight over 12 months without the struggle? The first way you'd probably have to gut it through the first month, and you're not likely to succeed in the next 11 months. The gradual way, you won't have cravings, so will be comfortable from the start.

Details

My approach to cut through all the dietary confusion is following what I call the "healthy eating" rules. .

1. Eat what everybody agrees you should eat: lots of whole or minimally processed foods like fruits and veggies, nuts, seeds, avocados, etc.
2. Avoid eating the stuff everybody agrees is bad for you-processed junk (especially refined carbs like soda, candy, cookies, etc.).
3. For foods that the experts or different diets disagree on, if you're concerned about any of them, just eat them in moderation.

As for rule #3, Dr. Michael Gregor, author of the excellent book <u>How Not To Die</u>, came up with another useful way of looking at borderline or controversial foods that is valid regardless of which diet you are following: the traffic light test[55].

There are "green" foods (eat plenty of these), "yellow" foods (eat in moderation), and "red" foods (avoid). By rule 2, anything everybody agrees is bad is red, while anything controversial (rule 3) is yellow. Most of us don't get enough green foods, so if a yellow food (like some minimally processed oil in your salad dressing) gets you to eat more green foods, that's a good thing.

You can really stress yourself out if you worry about the fine points too much about good and bad foods. There's actually a scientific term for this: orthorexia. Being relaxed about eating is probably better for your health than getting all the details right. So when in doubt, the 3 rules are a fallback.

You'll notice there is no mention of carb or fat content in the "healthy eating" rules. There has been much confusion generated by arguing about whether high carb/low fat or low carb/high fat is better. There are two reasons this misses the point. What is really important is to eat whole foods and avoid overly processed foods. It doesn't matter if it is high carb junk or low carb junk, it's still junk. There are good carbs (which is basically most carbs from whole or minimally processed plant sources) and good fats.

Which fats are good and bad is a bit controversial, and is discussed in the appendix, when in doubt that's what rule 3 is for. Second, the amount of carbs vs fats is not "one size fits all". As long as you're sticking to whole foods, and getting adequate but not excessive protein, there are a range of carb and fat levels that different people thrive on.

I describe a way to find out the best carb level for yourself in the section "resetting your metabolism". There are various diets that fit into the healthy eating guidelines if done properly, including wfpb, vegan, Mediterranean, paleo, and low-carb. While some of these can seem to be diametrically opposed, there is actually quite a bit of overlap among them. But you will still find disagreement, so when in doubt just remember the 3rd rule.

I do cover these diets in more detail below ("Details About Various Diets, and Health and Longevity Aspects"). Wfpb is more flexible than commonly thought, it does not have to be vegan, just reduced animal products, and can be readily "tuned" from higher carb/lower-fat to moderately low carb/higher fat. Both the vegan and Mediterranean diets can also be made subsets of wfpb. The paleo diet is also flexible- it can have various levels of meat consumption, as well as carb levels. As long as consumption of grains is reduced (especially if you have digestive intolerance to them), it is still paleo.

We'll see that a major role for low-carb diets is short term, in eliminating cravings. But a low or moderately low carb diet can also be formulated, and followed longer term, that follows the guidelines above.

Sticking to any kind of good diet can be easier said than done, especially since we are often more driven by cravings than rational decisions. It turns out these cravings have valid biological causes and will go away once you're eating "clean", it is not just about willpower. But if you just go straight to whole foods you may have to "gut out" having cravings while your metabolism fixes itself.

To shorten that unpleasant period, there are transition programs with sound science behind them, like that described in <u>Always Hungry?</u> This can eliminate cravings more quickly, and leave you in a position to effortlessly and enjoyably follow a good diet. At least, that's how it worked out for me, and 237 people in a pilot study of Dr Ludwig's program. I discuss Dr. Ludwig's approach below under "resetting your metabolism", along with a simplified version of it that I used. After doing this reset, you are in a good position to decide for yourself what's best for you (such as how many carbs can be in your diet without having any cravings, and what your tolerance is for some potential problem foods).

The Biology of Cravings in a Nutshell

Cravings have some strong biological origins. There are hormones like leptin and ghrelin that are supposed to control our hunger and match it to our bodies needs for calories. But they are thrown off by eating our overly processed, extremely calorie dense, modern diet.

The biological basis of cravings is discussed in detail in Dr. David Ludwig's book <u>Always Hungry?</u>, which goes to the heart of the matter of eliminating food cravings. I am summarizing his discussion here. One of the reasons for the out of whack hormones is that our fat cells become inflamed, or "angry" to use Dr. Ludwig's phrase. Fat is active tissue which plays a role in hormone signaling, and angry fat send the wrong messages.

This is made worse by not enough physical activity. The majority of Americans are sedentary, overweight or obese, with a high incidence of insulin resistance, or a more serious progression to type II diabetes. This situation is also occurring in many other countries who are increasingly following a modern diet of highly processed food.

Refined (or "bad") carbs are a major culprit because they cause a spike in blood sugar, which the body responds to by overproducing insulin, as shown in this figure from Dr. Ludwig's book[193].

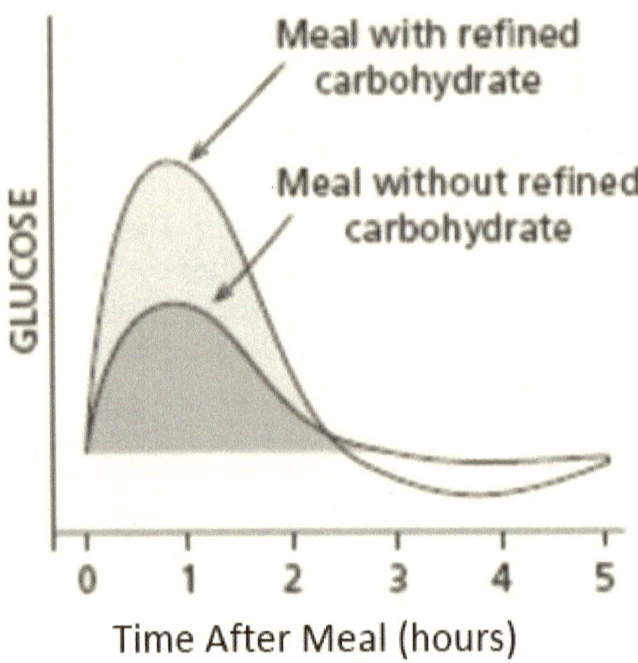

This sugar spike effect is often pointed out by various advocates of low-carb diets, but unfortunately they often fail to distinguish between refined and unrefined carbs when discussing this. It was also discussed by Dr. Terry Shintani in his book <u>The Good Carbohydrate Revolution</u>. An important thing to note is that, for the meal with bad carbs, glucose levels go below their original value before eating. This is called "rebound hypoglycemia", and leads to hunger cravings, often for more junk food.

Your brain can actually think this is an emergency situation because it won't be getting enough fuel if your blood sugar goes too low, so it pumps out adrenalin. No wonder we get in-between meal cravings. You're probably going to have trouble fighting off a snack after about two hours or so, and maybe want doughnuts midmorning or "grab a snickers" midafternoon. This will lead to another spike in blood glucose, so the process will start all over again.

Dr. Ludwig explains other deleterious effects on your metabolism in detail, including inflamed fat cells and bad effects on the hormones controlling hunger. I highly recommend reading his book for the fascinating account of how all this works (and for the solution to the problem). It's also important to point out that these effects, including inflamed fat cells, can occur in normal weight people (who can still have excess belly fat) as well as overweight people[179].

Losing and Maintaining Weight- Set Point, Palatability, Satiety, and Sustainability

Fat doesn't make you fat. Carbs don't make you fat. Overeating makes you fat. So what makes us overeat? The main culprit is modern processed food. Food companies actually try to find the "bliss point" in foods, the right combination of sugar, salt, and fat that will make you want to eat more[108]. Remember the Lays potato chip commercial: "I'll bet you can't eat just one"? They weren't kidding.

These foods have been shown to light up the pleasure centers in your brain like drugs[108]. Unfortunately they make up a lot of the SAD. This type of food isn't just unnaturally palatable (sometimes referred to as "hyperpalatable" in the literature[49]), it has an excessively high "food reward" which makes it taste like more. It's important instead to eat whole foods, which can still have plenty of flavor (palatability), but not excess "pleasure center" stimulation.

And food needs to promote satiety: after eating till pleasantly full, you should not be hungry again until several hours later. Finding a combination of good tasting whole foods that leaves you satisfied while consuming the right number of calories is the key. This is another reason to prefer whole foods over processed foods, because whole foods have much greater satiety[219]. Eating them will not make you feel deprived while losing weight, and is sustainable long term.

Satiety is a science of its own, that entire books are devoted to. One aspect is eating a diet that is nutritionally dense but not calorically dense, as proposed by Dr. Joel Fuhrman in <u>Eat To Live</u>[47]. If you eat broccoli till full, you'll have taken in a lot less calories than if you ate french fries till full. High fiber whole foods take up more room in your stomach and activate stretch receptors to send the full signal, which is the main point of the book <u>Volumetrics</u> by satiety researcher Dr. Barbara Rolls. Protein also has higher satiety. So eating lots of whole foods and adequate protein is a good way to make sure you get full without taking in too many calories.

Calories in vs calories out and the "set point"

Is there any truth to calories in vs calories out? If you eat more calories than you burn, you gain weight. If you eat less calories than you burn, you lose weight. Yes, it's just physics, and it has been proven many times in metabolic ward studies, where calories in and calories out are strictly controlled and measured.

But we don't live in metabolic wards, so there are complications. This is discussed at length in the book <u>The Calorie Myth</u> by Jonathan Bailor. Calories in can change calories out in a couple of ways. Your body has mechanisms to fight weight loss by defending your current weight ("set point"). The other effect is cravings, which make it hard to control calories in.

But is "a calorie is a calorie" true? Is 100 calories of candy the same as 100 calories of broccoli or 100 calories of eggs? There'd be two reasons to say no. The first is if they differ in the amount of cravings they cause. The second would be if there were some difference in the way they were metabolized in your body. It is controversial whether carbs, protein, of fats have a "metabolic advantage", which would mean you burn more calories eating say, 100 grams of protein vs 100 grams of carbs. Results from studies on this have been mixed, and the differences seen have been modest, so I'm going to ignore that effect for simplicity. That leaves the set point and cravings.

Different types of foods differ greatly in the cravings they can cause, as we just saw. Calories in vs calories out is not a useful concept unless cravings are under control. Otherwise it's Calories in → cravings → more calories in, leading to a vicious cycle.

Even if calories in vs calories out matters, that would not mean weight loss and maintenance is just a matter of willpower. I am disciplined enough to have trained for and run marathons. But I could still not control my eating enough not to get overweight. There are people that still struggle controlling their eating who are disciplined enough to be ultramarathoners running 100 mile races[127] or Ironman triathletes[162].

Another issue about calories in vs calories out is the "set point", discussed in detail in <u>Always Hungry?</u> and in <u>The Calorie Myth</u>. This is your body's tendency to "defend" it's current weight, which has survival advantages if calories are scarce. If your body thinks you are in danger of starving, it can compensate by hormonal changes that cause hunger, to try to force you to increase calories in. It can also turn down calories out by making you feel more fatigued so you'll move less, or turning down your metabolism, for example, with hormones that affect the thyroid[179].

There are misconceptions about the set point, such as that it is carved in stone or genetic, causing people to despair that they can ever lose weight. These are discussed in detail in Michael Fumento's book <u>Fat of the Land</u> about the obesity epidemic[195], where he dismisses the misconceptions as myths. The set point should be thought of as equivalent to the setting on a thermostat. Just like you can adjust the temperature on a thermostat, you can lower the set point to a new lower weight.

Exercising, losing weight gradually, eating minimally processed foods, and resetting your metabolism all help do that. But trying to lose weight too fast, especially by counting calories and intentionally cutting back on calories in, can trigger the "set point" effects and make it harder to succeed at losing weight and keeping it off.

The best approach is to do the metabolic reset described below, and after that, continuing on with "healthy eating" eating should allow you to eat till full, while bringing in the amount of calories your body needs. If you are overweight, that will automatically be somewhat less than needed to maintain your current weight, so gradual weight loss will occur. And your set point will slowly but surely lower to the new weight.

When you reach your target, your set point should now be at that weight, and rather than try to fight you to regain back to your previous weight, your body will happily maintain at the new level. If your metabolism is working properly, and you are eating minimally processed food, then counting calories should be unnecessary. If you eat till satisfied, your body's internal wisdom should work to send the "full" signal when you've eaten the right amount of calories. That's assuming you don't eat too fast, it can take 20 minutes for your brain to notice your stomach is full.

Good and Bad Carbs: Glycemic Index/Glycemic Load

Measuring the glucose vs time graph shown in the figure above allows us to determine how good or bad the carbs are in various foods by quantifying the "glucose spike". The amount of sugar in the blood two hours after ingesting 50 grams of a specific food is used to determine the glycemic index or GI (it's the area under the glucose vs time graph at 2 hours, for math nerds like me). So low GI is good, high is bad. GI works great for most foods, but is misleading for some, like carrots, for which 50g is a very large serving. So in my opinion glycemic load, or GL, is a better measure, because this factors in the number of carbs in the actual serving of food[187]. So the formal definition of a "good" carb is one with a low enough glycemic load, while a bad carb has high glycemic load. You could actually use a chart to check all your foods, but this would be tedious. I think it's enough to keep in mind what the potential problem foods might be, which are all refined foods, plus some starchy fruits and vegetables and some grains. White potatoes have a higher GL than sweet potatoes, for example.

When in doubt, for a borderline food, The Good Carbohydrate Revolution recommends keeping GL under 20, and has an extensive chart. It's still in print in paperback. There is also a list in Always Hungry?

It's not like you're going to fall off a cliff because you ate one baked potato. But If your cravings come back, maybe consider what you ate recently, and avoid or cut back on the likely culprit.

Resetting Your Metabolism

The obvious answer to all the metabolic issues caused by
eating refined carbs seems to be just get them out of your diet.
That was proposed in <u>The Good Carbohydrate Revolution</u>
and also by various wfpb diet proponents (dating way back to
Nathan Pritikin in 1979) and Paleo and low-carb authors. It
apparently works well for many people. In the figure above,
for the meal with no refined carbs, there is no rebound
hypoglycemia so there should be no cravings.

But when you first eliminate refined carbs, until your
metabolism is fixed, you're likely to have a period of cravings,
which you may have to "gut through" before you can sustain
this clean diet. To shorten this period, Dr. Ludwig proposes a
temporary eating period to reset your metabolism to normal,
including, as he puts it "calming your angry fat cells". I highly
recommend his book if you want to try it. I was going to
summarize it here but decided you really need to read the
book to get all the nuances. I'll describe my simplified version
here.

First let me point out that this is not the same as the "kick
start" that many diet books have. It's not "go through my one
month boot camp and lose 20 pounds to start you on your
weight loss journey". This is to fix your metabolism and you
may not have any weight loss at all at first. The first signs of
progress are instead starting to enjoy healthier foods and
reduced cravings for unhealthy foods.

The "kick start" mentality often fails because of the focus on weight loss. You start with a burst of enthusiasm and maybe get some motivation from initial positive results from the scale, but then get discouraged if the weight loss plateaus or slows down. Also, kickstarts as part of diets often involve calorie restriction, which leaves you physically hungry and will probably activate the body's set point mechanism with a vengeance. That's a tough fight to win.

The reset does not involve calorie deprivation, but instead substitutes eating till pleasantly full with healthier foods. These foods tend to be more satisfying so there's a good chance you'll get full on fewer calories, causing weight loss to gradually occur as a byproduct, but weight loss is not the focus during the reset. I did not follow Dr. Ludwig's program to the letter, but used a simplified approach that worked fine for me, that does not require counting carbs. I also had the insight that, after cravings are eliminated, you are in a good position to experiment with carb level, legume tolerance, etc., to tune the diet to what works best for you.

Here's my simple version:

- Be really strict about refined carbs, and limit starchy unrefined carbs like potatoes, during the reset. Eat all the minimally processed whole foods you want. If they don't provide enough calories to feel satisfied, eat more fat during this time. But it helps to avoid commercial vegetable oils and products made from them, because they have an inflammatory effect on the body, which doesn't help with healing the biological reasons for cravings. I used extra virgin olive oil (evoo) and organic expeller pressed canola oil. Good and bad fats are discussed in detail in the appendix.

- If you think you might have digestive sensitivities to grains or legumes, you can omit them during the reset.
- Follow this for a minimum of 2 weeks until cravings disappear completely (I was lucky so for me they diminished right away and were gone after about 3 weeks).

After the reset comes a transition period where you find out what works for you long term:

- If you have eliminated grains or legumes, I recommend reintroducing them and seeing if they cause digestive issues. Legumes should be first because they are an important source of nutrients including protein. Traditional cultures have reduced the digestive issues of legumes with foods like tofu and tempeh, so these, or meat substitutes based on them, are another alternative you may tolerate if you have a problem with legumes. If any of these foods do cause digestive problems you may be intolerant to them and need to leave them out.

- Next you can experiment with your carb level. You can introduce more starchy but low glycemic foods like sweet potatoes or bananas. I personally can also get away with them, and with white potatoes in moderation. All of these are upping the carb content of the diet. If at any time cravings return, back off. If you were not able to add too many carbs back in it means you are less carb tolerant, even for good carbs (carb tolerance is discussed below). That does not matter because you can still eat a variety of nutritious foods even if the diet stays moderately low carb, as long as you emphasize lots of fruits and veggies. You just may need to go easy on starchier foods. I did not measure the carbs vs fat when I did this, I just ate till satisfied with plenty of whole food sources of fat like nuts, seeds, avocados. When reintroducing starchy foods I did not cut back on whole food fat sources, but instead cut back on oils.
- If after reading the information on longevity and health aspects of animal foods in the appendix, you decide to cut back on animal foods, you can start experimenting with replacing some animal sources of protein with plant sources.

Hopefully after this reset/transition you will reconnect with your body's wisdom on how much to eat. You can eat a variety of delicious foods till satisfied, and gradually lose weight if necessary, after which weight management is much easier (because, as discussed under "calories in/calories out", your body's set point will lower itself to the new weight). And cravings will be totally gone. I discussed how it went for me above. I sincerely hope it works out that way for you too!

You've probably noted that following this reset and transition will involve giving up some old friends like soda and your favorite snacks, so it is going to be challenging. To face this challenge, it helps to fix your food environment, and address psychological and behavioral issues of cravings, as discussed next.
If the reset sounds too extreme for you, an alternative is the "mini-habits" approach of phasing in healthy eating, described below under "ditch the diet mentality".

Psychological, Behavioral, and Environmental Aspects of Cravings

Some people might not be as lucky as me, so cravings might not disappear right away when they start the "reset". And some people still have psychological cravings after the reset has fixed physical ones. There are psychological and behavioral techniques, at least some of which I'm sure you've encountered elsewhere if you've ever read any books on weight loss. I'll summarize a few that have worked for me:

- Fix your food environment. The front line of the battle against "off-plan" foods is in the store, not your house. It's harder to fight them once they are conveniently there in the house. But to win the fight in the store, you have to plan in advance, have a list, and stick to it. In <u>Salt, Sugar, and Fat</u>, Michael Moss cites the statistic that, on average, 70% of food purchases are unplanned[108]. The food industry is well aware of that, which is why there are tempting displays as you enter the store and on "end caps". You'll never see artfully arranged broccoli in such a display, more likely chips and dip or beer.

- Eat slowly. The stomach notices right away when it is getting full because it has stretch receptors, but it can take the brain about 20 minutes to respond to the signal from the stomach. If you are eating fast you can pack in a lot more calories before the brain flips the "full" switch.

- Eat mindfully (paying attention). No fussing with a smartphone or computer or watching TV, we occasionally need a break from all of that anyway. My most enjoyable meals are paying 100% attention to my food plus my friends or loved ones. I must admit I don't do this all the time. I might eat at my desk sometimes while eating breakfast and mindlessly shove food in my face, and then be disappointed when I notice it's gone already.

- Control stress: eating when you're stressed out more likely leads to making the wrong food choices.

There are many books devoted solely to this topic. An interesting one is <u>Mindless Eating: Why We Eat More Than We Think</u> by Dr. Brian Wansink, who has done a lot of research on this, including in a fascinating restaurant where the patrons on one side form the control group and those on the other the experimental group. Tidbits from the book include: if told to eat as much as we want, we tend to eat more food if given a larger full plate vs a smaller one. Moviegoers given free popcorn will eat more if given a larger size container, even if the popcorn is stale. In a companion book <u>Slim by Design: Mindless Eating Solutions for Everyday Life</u>, he gives tips on how to control our food environment at home and our choices when eating out, to reduce the mindless overeating we tend to do. One simple example: having a fruit bowl out in plain sight tends to double the amount of fruit we eat.

Ditch The "Going On A Diet" Mentality

I mentioned above that I don't believe in "going on a diet" but didn't say why. The problem is it has a very low success rate in the long run. You can make progress in the short term but then almost inevitably "lose it" and gain the weight back. In his book <u>Mini Habits for Weight Loss</u>, Stephen Guise goes over this in great detail and gives a lot of scientific evidence why it doesn't work. There's much psychological insight in this recommended book.

Instead of the going on a diet mentality, he suggests, as I do, the attitude of making a long term change to a healthier way of eating. His approach to do so is interesting and psychologically sound: Mini habits. These are small changes that are easy to make, and you can succeed at. I mentioned Stephen's ideas on using this approach for physical activity. In this book, he shows how it works for eating also, like start out eating one extra piece of fruit per day.

The idea is to make small easy changes that you can be successful at, which gradually leads to more change, and eventually enjoying your new healthier behaviors. As discussed below under "Physical Activity and Weight Loss", it's a bit controversial whether to try to change your eating habits and your physical activity simultaneously. But Stephen definitely feels it works well in the context of mini-habits, because they are small changes that don't overly strain your willpower.

So you could, for example, readily do the mini-habit of one extra piece of fruit a day while at the same time adding a habit of getting up from your desk to take a NEAT break more often. The mini-habits approach can be used as a supplement to use to address psychological cravings after the reset has fixed physical ones. That worked well for me.

But if you think the reset sounds too drastic and are concerned about having the willpower to make it through it, mini-habits offer also a more slow and steady alternative to the reset. Using them you gradually introduce some healthy foods to your diet, which eventually becomes an established behavior, and starts to displace unhealthy foods. This should also over time make your diet more anti-inflammatory and start to address the biological aspects of cravings. I think a good place to start for folks my age would be a mini-habit to eat more berries and walnuts, since these appear to support good brain health as well as other benefits[232, 233].

The 80/20 Rule and "Cheating"

Most advocates of any diet think it is ok if you eat "on-plan" about 80% of the time. So what is the 20% for? Partly it is the idea I discussed above about using "yellow" foods to make "green" foods more enjoyable, such as using oils in salad dressings even though they are not whole foods. Or to allow some bread every once in a while at a restaurant or dessert at a party. I like to think of it as there are no forbidden foods, but some foods are "staples of your diet", while others are occasional "special treats".

But some authors go so far as to allow "cheat" meals or "cheat" days, which can be a bad idea psychologically. To be sustainable, your way of eating has to be enjoyable, you can't be thinking of it as deprivation and straying from it as fun. An obvious example is the mindset of being "good" on weekdays while getting to have "fun" on weekends. First of all, the weekend is 29% of the week, so that exceeds your 20% budget, but more importantly it can lead to more severe "straying" than a piece of bread or cake, especially if alcohol gets into the picture.

Rob Wolf objects to the idea of "cheating" because it implies we're being immoral, and devotes an entire chapter to this in <u>Wired To Eat</u>[163]. This can cause all kinds of psychological problems, like "in for a penny in for a pound": "I cheated. I'm a failure, I may as well go for it and have a real binge" or even worse, give up on trying to change my way of eating. If you occasionally eat "off-plan", just get "back on the wagon" at your next meal.

There is an interesting idea for going off-plan in a controlled way for endurance athletes in <u>The Paleo Diet for Athletes</u> by Dr. Loren Cordain and Joe Friel. Coach Friel suggests allowing yourself to eat more carbs, even refined carbs, after a long workout. This helps psychologically because it gives you a reward to look forward to after a challenging session, and it's also physiologically the least harmful time to stray.

After a long workout you've depleted the glycogen levels in your muscles and your body will take the carbs you eat afterwards and send them right off to replenish your muscle stores. I'm talking about after a tough workout of 90 minutes or so, not a 30 minute walk. This is also something I would not consider doing until you've already gone through the reset, because you want to be sure you are not insulin resistant.

His suggestion is actually controversial because some coaches feel it may interfere with optimal training adaptations. But I think that is an issue more for competitive athletes, and for amateurs like me it is less important. I implemented Coach Friel's suggestion on the day of my longest workout (ride, hike, or combination), which may be about 2 to 3 hours, and is in the morning. I don't eat a lot of carbs at breakfast beforehand and don't take in calories during the workout. Afterwards I occasionally allow myself some refined carbs (even soda!) which would normally be way off limits. But this is just for one meal a week.

Outsmarting The Hungry Brain

Neurologist and obesity expert Dr. Stephan Guyenet wrote an interesting book The Hungry Brain[194] which shows how our brains are wired to overeat in the presence of abundant calories. He also tells a story that's a fascinating reason for us to avoid eating junk. Obesity researchers studying rats needed a dependable way to get them to gain weight. If they were fed rat chow spiked with extra sugar or extra fat, they would overeat and gain weight, but not as quickly or reliably as hoped. Then someone who'd been snacking on froot loops tried giving some to the rats. They went crazy for them, overeating like mad. The researchers then tried various processed food items which got dubbed the "cafeteria diet", similar to the processed main course foods and treats you could get at a cafeteria. They all worked great. So when you are eating junk, you are eating food that's works well to fatten up a rat as quickly as possible. Unfortunately, it's also effective for fattening up humans.

Dr. Guyenet Recommends six steps for outsmarting your hungry brain:

- Fix your food environment- we discussed this one above.
- Let your brain know you aren't starving- eat high satiety foods that are palatable but not overly so- we discussed that above under "losing and maintaining weight- set point, palatability, satiety, sustainability".
- Beware of high "food reward" (hyperpalatable food) - another reason for whole foods, no junk.
- Get good quality sleep- He cites research showing that sleep-deprived people may overeat by 300 calories per day.
- Physical activity- exercise in moderation helps create a calorie deficit without triggering the "set point", and there's some evidence it slowly lowers the set point over time.
- Stress- we tend to overeat and make poor food choices when under stress. I discuss stress management in chapter 5.

Physical Activity and Weight Loss

One of the big debates you'll see is whether physical activity is beneficial for weight loss. The reasoning is usually based on calories in vs. calories out: "if you walk for half an hour you might burn 150 calories. You take in more than that by eating one doughnut". My first thought is "Uh, don't eat the doughnut?" But I also think this argument is missing the main benefits of exercise, which go beyond calorie burning. It has various overall health benefits discussed in the appendix, as well as several for weight loss besides calorie burning:

- It decreases insulin resistance[7], by various mechanisms, one of which is an improvement in density and function of mitochondria (the energy powerhouses in our cells that help us use oxygen)[102, 87, 57]. Less IR means less cravings, making it easier to adhere to a better diet.
- Resistance training and higher intensity exercise can raise resting metabolic rate for a prolonged period after the training is over[14, 70].
- All types of exercise can reduce the decline in resting metabolic rate that accompanies weight loss[9].
- Resistance training helps preserve muscle mass during weight loss[69].
- Being physically active can help lower the body's metabolic set point over time, allowing a lower weight to be maintained[194].

How much you should exercise while also trying to change your way of eating is controversial. Many authors feel that if you are already active, fine, keep up what you are doing, but now would not be a good time to introduce a new exercise routine. The idea is that we only have so much willpower and would be dividing it up between being disciplined about what you are eating and disciplined about exercising.

There is some counter evidence to this, however, that showed greater long term success for people modifying their eating habits while simultaneously modifying their physical activity compared to those who modified their eating first and only added physical activity a few months later[220]. I would suspect this to be especially true for resistance training and HIIT based on the evidence in the appendix on "the anti-aging and metabolic benefits of resistance training and HIIT".

I think it's a good idea to at least work on bumping up NEAT through your activities of daily living while working on healthier eating. It will get you some of the metabolic benefits of being active without requiring as much discipline.

I have always been physically active any time I tried to lose weight or change my eating, so I can't comment from experience on trying to start a new exercise program while also trying to change my eating habits. But I do know from experience about the trap of thinking of exercise primarily as a way of burning calories. I have exercised a sensible amount that's enjoyable for me, say an hour a day, with mostly easy days and a couple of hard days thrown in. Then maybe I would do well on the scale that week. The lesson should have been, you're doing fine, keep up the good work. Instead I'd get excited and say, "Wow I could do even better if I worked out more! I'll burn a couple more thousand calories next week by exercising longer and throwing in some more hard days". The next week I'd either slip up on my eating discipline and not lose any weight, or get discouraged because I was disciplined about eating and exercise but lost less than I expected. One time, I carefully measured everything I ate, and worked out for over 90 minutes a day. At the end of the week I got discouraged because I "only" lost 2½ pounds! This is all short-term thinking, similar to the mindset of "being on a diet". The long view, for both eating and physical activity, works better: Exercise is for healthy aging and a good metabolism, not to make the needle move on the scale.

Carb Tolerance

Theoretically, after the reset, with a properly functioning metabolism, you should be able to eat as many carbs as you want as long as they are good carbs (unrefined and not high glycemic). Some authors, especially of low-carb diets, argue that a lot of people are carb intolerant and need fewer carbs, even good carbs, in the long term.

They assume that if you are currently overweight or have any signs of insulin resistance, it means you are genetically intolerant to all carbs. That makes it hard to explain how the population of the US was a lot leaner in 1900 even though they ate a similar percentage of carbs compared to today (folks ate the same percentage of carbs then, but a lot less bad carbs, except for white bread)[51].

There are also two populations that disprove the assumption about genetic intolerance to all carbs: Hawaiians on their original high carb diet were very fit and trim, as reported by early westerners that visited them. The exception were the nobility, who had access to richer foods, and sometimes became obese. Hawaiians on a modern diet have a major problem with obesity and metabolic issues. Yet they can readily lose weight and become healthy if they go back to their traditional diet, which is high in minimally processed carbs (including a lot of taro root)[144].

The other example is the Native American Pima tribe. They traditionally ate a high carb, wfpb diet, very low in animal products, and were slender and healthy. The branch of the tribe on the Mexican side of the border retained their traditional lifestyle and diet along with its good health. Unfortunately, on the US side in Arizona, the Pima were forced off their land onto a reservation and adopted our western diet. They have much higher incidences of diabetes and obesity than the US average, indicating they may have some genetic difference that makes the modern diet extra harmful to them. But an effort has been made to reintroduce the traditional diet to Arizona Pimas, and it has led to remarkable health improvements and weight loss[129]. I would argue that both these populations more likely have a genetically low tolerance for *bad* carbs, not *all* carbs.

Carb tolerance, even if it has a genetic component, is probably not "carved in stone". The "metabolic reset" should improve it, as will losing weight. Adding physical activity if you are sedentary is also known to improve it. There are healthy populations that eat up to 80% carbs described in the appendix. They are all very physically active.

As a final note, there is some evidence for different levels of genetic tolerance for starch as discussed in the appendix under "Paleolithic Nutrition". So some people, whose ancestors probably leaned more towards "gatherer" than hunter, may be able to eat all they want of starchy vegetables like potatoes, and starchy fruits like bananas, while others may need to consume these more moderately but can still eat all they want of non-starchy carbs.

You can find out for yourself what your carb tolerance is during the transition. As long as the level of good carbs you are eating does not cause cravings to return, you are fine.

Narrow Eating Window

This is a health promoting technique that can be used with any diet. Simply avoiding evening snacking causes a fast each night until we break that fast the next morning, which is where the name breakfast comes from. If you finish dinner at 6 PM and don't eat until breakfast at 8 AM the next morning, all your eating takes place in a 10 hour "window" from 8 AM till 6 PM, and you do a mini-fast the other 14 hours.

This is the simplest form of "intermittent fasting", which has been promoted as a weight loss technique. But I think its main benefit is for general health: it allows the body to enter a cleanup stage (apoptosis and autophagy) where cellular waste is recycled and cells that are no longer useful are removed[137].

Details About Various Diets, and Health and Longevity Aspects

At the end of the reset you are eating a moderately low-carb diet and it is time to find out the best long-term way of eating for you in the transition. I go over the health aspects of various diet alternatives in this section. There is some controversy about what I am about to cover, even though I tried to present balanced evidence and look for what's in common among various approaches. Far and away the biggest takeaway on diet is just following the "healthy eating rules", rather than any specific detail that might be controversial.

Wfpb (Whole Foods Plant Based) diet

A whole foods plant based diet gets a reduced percentage of its calories from animal products, the rest from a variety of healthy plant foods. There are data on healthy and long-lived populations around the world that eat this way (it is the only diet for which we have population data showing improved longevity).

In addition to the population data, there are also intervention studies showing wfpb can reverse heart disease[115,37], including the Ornish and Esselstyn studies discussed in the appendix. These were hospital based studies, but a community-based program using the wfpb diet was developed by Dr. Howard Diehl, called the Coronary Health Improvement Program, and was also shown to have great success on thousands of participants with heart diseases and other diseases. It was so effective on other conditions, and for weight loss, that it was renamed the Community Health Improvement Program and is still in use today. It has been described as "achieving some of the most impressive clinical outcomes published in the literature"[210], for its clinical benefits as well as cost-effectiveness. So why haven't we heard of it? Wouldn't it be nice if news like this were trumpeted by the media instead of the latest fad?

Carbs vs. fat in the wfpb diet can be adjusted quite a bit by trading grains and starchy fruits and vegetables for higher fat foods like nuts, seeds, and avocados. So it can be used during the reset and even can be used as a moderately low carb diet. For people who are intolerant of either grains or legumes, consumption of them can be reduced. For example, one of the healthy populations mentioned above is the Ikarians, who consume only 4% of their calories from grains and 7% from legumes. In this form, wfpb is similar to a lower-meat version of paleo.

Some people thrive on wfpb right away, others (like me) may need to do a "reset" first to get their metabolism in line and avoid cravings. To learn more about the specifics of the wfpb diet, I recommend <u>How Not to Die</u>, by Dr. Michael Gregor, and <u>Eat to Live</u>, by Dr. Joel Fuhrman. There is also a wealth of science-based nutritional info on Dr. Gregor's website www.nutritionfacts.org.

Vegan

The vegan, or 100% plant food, diet is a subset of wfpb if it is properly formulated. There are many foods that are vegan that are not whole foods, like oreos, soda, french fries, and beer. A vegan diet that includes a significant amount of foods like those is poorly formulated and is not recommended. But the vegan version of wfpb is healthy, as exemplified by Seventh Day Adventist vegans, who are among the healthiest populations in the world[114].

Mediterranean

The Mediterranean diet is patterned after by the eating habits
of Greece, southern Italy, and Spain in the 1950s[183], and
includes high consumption of olive oil, legumes, unrefined
grains, fruits, and vegetables, moderate consumption of fish,
dairy products (mostly as cheese and yogurt), and wine, and
low consumption of non-fish meat foods[183]. Modern followers
of it get up to 70% of their grain consumption from refined
grains, which have a relatively high glycemic load[39], and this
does not fit in with wfpb.

Also, many people have the misconception that olive oil is
what makes the Mediterranean diet healthy, and they can just
indiscriminately pour it on their food. As discussed in the
appendix under "controversial fats", even extra virgin olive
oil should be used in moderation. There are authors proposing
health improvements to the Mediterranean diet[40] that reduce
consumption of the foods that are not whole foods, and in this
form it is a subset of wfpb.

Low Fat

Some wfpb authors like Dr. Caldwell Esselstyn[37] and Dr. John McDougall[184] advocate tuning wfpb to the low end of fat content. Dr Esselstyn promotes the low-fat version because his primary concern is reversing heart disease. If you already have symptoms of heart disease like angina, the low fat version of wfpb might be a good idea for you. Other people, who are highly carb tolerant (typically those who are lean and fit), may also thrive on this version. Dr. Dean Ornish points out in his book <u>The Spectrum</u> that people who are not trying to reverse heart disease, but want to eat healthy to reduce risk of heart disease and other conditions, can afford to loosen up on the amount of fat.

Low fat is a disaster if done improperly, especially if you are eating lots of refined carbs. But low fat has an advantage if you are eating good carbs and are carb tolerant, so it does not cause cravings: It is nutrient dense but not calorically dense. You can get full, and get a lot of nutrition without eating a lot of calories. This was the point of Dr. Dean Ornish's <u>Eat More Weigh Less</u>[116]. This only works with good carbs, as the US population should now be well aware, having gone through a low-fat era where many people thought it was ok to eat all the pretzels, cookies, and ice cream they wanted as long as they were low fat.

Paleo

This diet is based on evidence that traditional pre-agricultural populations were robust and healthy compared to people in agricultural civilizations (see "Paleolithic Nutrition"). Hunter gatherers ate a variety of plant foods plus animal foods like meat and fish, but little or no dairy.

The version of paleo often presented is relatively high in consumption of animal products (except dairy). Many people do well on this version, but it does bring up the long-term health concerns discussed in the appendix for meat and excessive protein consumption (which, admittedly, may be controversial). But some paleo authors are less rigid in their interpretation. For example, paleo author Rob Wolf has a new book <u>Wired To Eat</u> on the subject of personalized nutrition, and argues that paleo is not "one size fits all". In this flexible form, paleo is more like "no dairy, minimal grains, reduced legumes".

If you find you can tolerate and enjoy legumes, or some legume-based products like meat substitutes, then it is straightforward to dial back the percentage of calories from animal products in the paleo diet and replace some of them with legume-based foods. This can even be done without legumes with some non-grain, non-legume foods that are high in protein like buckwheat (which is neither wheat nor a grain, it's a seed) and mushrooms. I recommend Rob Wolf's <u>Wired To Eat</u> as a start for more information on a flexible paleo diet, especially if you think you might have intolerance to grains or legumes.

I suspect that one of the main reasons people do well on paleo is that a lot of our favorite modern processed treats contain grains or dairy (such as cake, cookies, ice cream, pretzels) so right away paleo is making you cut back on them. It is still important to stay away from other processed foods, of course. Even if you can argue that our ancestors could have ground corn or sliced potatoes and cooked them in fat, that doesn't make it a good idea to eat "o" foods, like potato chips, fritos, doritos, etc.

Low Carb

Proponents of low-carb diets aggressively try to minimize blood glucose spikes. They emphasize eating good carbs, as does wfpb, but argue that there is additional benefit if all carbs are restricted. The main reason presented is that carbs, especially bad carbs, can cause a blood glucose spike leading to metabolic problems as well as cravings and overeating, as discussed above. In my opinion, the most important use of low-carb is as a short-term reset to our metabolisms to eliminate these cravings as we saw above.

But as discussed above under "carb tolerance", it is not clear that keeping all carbs low is necessary long term for most people, as long as their metabolisms have been "reset" and bad carbs are avoided. We also saw you can find this out for yourself after the reset.

In the last 20 years or so, a significant amount of research has been done on the health and effectiveness of low-carb diets, and various short-term metabolic health benefits have been found[46,98,157]. There are no population or observational studies showing long-term health benefits for this diet, as discussed in detail in the appendix.

Some long term studies showed low carb was associated with significantly increased risk of all-cause mortality if the diet was animal-based (emphasizing animal sources of fat and protein), but had a decreased risk of mortality if it was vegetable-based (emphasizing vegetable sources of fat and protein)[48, 146]. Long term low carb is also associated with increased risk of type II diabetes, but again only if the diet is high in fat and protein from animal foods[23]. If a moderately low carb diet emphasizes plant sources of fat and protein, it is equivalent to wfpb.

Ketogenic

The ketogenic (or "keto") diet is popular right now. You can see signs proclaiming foods to be "keto friendly" in grocery stores. I think the main reason is it can be an effective weight loss approach. Ketogenic diets intentionally keep carbs very low to induce ketosis, a survival mechanism the body uses to supply fuel to the brain when not enough total calories or calories from carbs are available in the diet- the brain cannot use fat as fuel, it can only use glucose or the alternative fuel "ketone bodies". Ketosis is called nutritional ketosis when it is intentionally induced by a diet, and such diets are called ketogenic.

The term "ketogenic diet" was coined by Dr Russel Wilder, at the Mayo Clinic, who first used it in 1921 to treat patients with epilepsy[189]. It still plays a useful role for that purpose and for some other clinical conditions[62]. A lot of the benefits claimed for the keto diet are common with non-keto low carb or a moderately-low-carb reset.

There are many short term benefits for it discussed in <u>The Art and Science of Low-Carbohydrate Living</u> by Drs Jeff Volek and Stephen Phinney, who have done pioneering research on this diet. But while impressive, the studies are almost always in comparison to either the SAD or a low fat diet that is not whole food plant based. And unfortunately, the authors often do not distinguish between good and bad carbs in their discussions. This makes it difficult to discern what the unique benefits of the ketogenic diet might be.

The most famous diet that uses ketosis is the Atkins diet, and it only uses it short term (2 weeks) for its induction phase. This is actually quite similar to a reset and transition. In the induction phase you are in ketosis, which functions like a reset to your metabolism, then you add a bit more good carbs back in, and stay in a non-ketogenic low carb phase while losing weight. After reaching your goal weight, you gradually add more carbs, stopping if any weight gain occurs[171].

Some aspects of the original Atkins diet, like allowing liberal amounts of saturated fat and processed meats, are still controversial. But the diet can be followed while avoiding those controversial foods, and after the short term induction it could be followed in a form that reduces consumption of animal products (in this form it has been referred to as "eco-Atkins"[234]). This is more similar to wfpb tuned to the lower end of the carb spectrum.

It is possible not everyone will respond to a moderately low carb reset as presented in this book and in Always Hungry? Perhaps if your metabolism is more severely dysfunctional it would need a "bigger hammer" to get it back on track, and following short term keto as in the Atkins diet may function well for that purpose.

But I believe the percentage of the population that might need that is much smaller than most proponents of the ketogenic diet assume, as was discussed above under carb tolerance. More recent authors are proposing using the ketogenic diet for a much longer period[121]. Exaggerated claims are also made that this diet is needed, long term, for a large percentage of adults, which was disproved above under "carb tolerance".

The idea that a dysfunctional metabolism could be healed by a temporary fix like the reset, or short term use of ketosis, seems to be neglected by such authors. They discuss followers of the diet "losing it" when transitioning to a higher level of carbs in their diets. That is certainly a danger for bad carbs, but it is hard to fathom that many people would not be able to handle a moderately low-carb, non-ketogenic diet, with the carbs consisting only of good carbs, without experiencing cravings. However, if you use the ketogenic diet for weight loss, and then transition out of it, I agree it's vital to realize this is a tricky period and to diligently avoid bad carbs during this time.

In addition to the health aspects about low-carb diets in general discussed above, there is some long-term evidence of deleterious effects specifically of the ketogenic diet. Most of these studies are on patients being treated over a long period (multiple years) for epilepsy with the diet. Adverse effects include signs of vascular damage and increased arterial stiffness[211], cardiac complications[212], and symptoms of bone demineralization (Increased risk of kidney stones and high calcium levels in the blood)[128].

The concern of doing this diet wrong is high because it is "in" right now, and less qualified authors are jumping on the bandwagon. Two important caveats are: make sure to spend your limited carb budget on healthy foods like greens and berries, and take steps to keep the diet alkaline. This is discussed in detail on Dr. Anna Cabeca's website: http://drannacabeca.com/kick-start-a-new-keto-alkaline-you/.

Chapter 5- The Other Pillars of Health: Social Support and Stress Management

Social Support

When you read about the healthy and long-lived populations such as in the Blue Zones, discussed in the appendix, yes they eat a good diet. But they are also quite active physically and have strong social support, both from their extended families and their communities. Getting together with friends and family, dancing, and singing, are all frequent parts of their daily lives.

Dr. Dean Ornish, who did the famous study on reversing heart disease, readily admits that his program is a package deal, and that social support is at least as important as diet. He chronicles this in the moving book <u>Love and Survival</u>, which talks about the members of the support groups associated with the program. Some of them had terminal cancer but lived longer and better because of their participation in their groups, which became a loving extended family.

We are drifting too much towards isolation in the modern world, a trend we need to fight. Family and extended family is a good place to start, even if long distances intervene. I already mentioned some ways to turn physical activity into social support.

Churches and meditation groups are another example, and all sorts of groups with common interest can be found on the meetup site (www.meetup.com). These are ways to find like-minded people to meet with in person. Facebook, instagram, and other "social media" don't count, in my opinion.

Purpose in Life

Having a purpose in life is strongly related to longevity. Okinawan elders have a saying for this that roughly translates "what do you get up for in the morning?"[178] Many people get this from their careers and can lose it after retirement. But there are plenty of other ways, including family, hobbies, lifelong learning (through books, adult ed or many online courses now available), and volunteer work. One doctor suggested that the answer to the question "do you volunteer" was the most important predictor of continued health in his older patients.

A researcher came up with an assessment test for purpose in life in older people, and correlated the results with risk for dementia. Those who scored 4.2 out of 5 or higher on the test were 2.4 times more likely to remain free of dementia than those who scored a 3 or less[8].

Stress Management

Stress in our modern world is every bit as much of a health risk as poor diet. Physical activity and social support both go a long way towards relieving it. There are also some formal mental techniques which help quite a bit.

Mindfulness

This is just paying attention to what is going on in the present moment, something modern society seems to be moving away from more and more these days. Many of the people I see when I'm out walking are fussing with their phones. Aside from the danger of walking into a pole, they are missing out on their often beautiful surroundings. I even saw this recently in Yosemite Valley, one of the most picturesque places I know, where people were walking the foot paths staring at their phones.

You see entire families in restaurants eating and playing with their phones, none of them paying attention to each other. One of the saddest examples I saw recently was a woman who had taken her two young toddlers to the park and put them on the swings. She'd give one a push, mess around with the phone for a while, then give the other a push, and kept alternating that way. Once in a while she'd get lost in the phone and forget to push either kid until one would yell "Mom!" and she'd reluctantly drag herself back away from the phone. She sounds like a good candidate to take the "smartphone compulsion test" (http://virtual-addiction.com/smartphone-compulsion-test) or read Catherine Price's book How to Break Up with Your Phone[124].

In his book <u>The Brain Warrior's Way</u>, Dr. Daniel Amen cites evidence that the average attention span in the US has shrunk from an already poor 12 seconds in 2000 to a pitiful 8 seconds now. If the same test is applied to goldish, they outscore us by lasting 9 seconds. I don't think our species is evolving in the right direction with this trend.

Here's how I first found out about mindfulness. The most stressful time in my life was when I was working at a startup. We had a lot of difficult work to do and were often in a time crunch. But we were using workstations with multiple windows. What a productivity tool! I could work on several things at once, while a piece of code was compiling in one window (which could take a couple of minutes back in the 80s and early 90s), I could work on something else in another. I felt tremendously productive. But I noticed after a while that some of the tasks on my todo list today were to fix something I screwed up previously, maybe because of being distracted by a second thing I was working on. Maybe this isn't all so productive after all.

Then I read <u>The Miracle of Mindfulness</u> by the Vietnamese Buddhist monk and great teacher Thich Nhat Hanh, about the value of doing one thing at a time, and always paying 100% attention to what you are doing. So I closed down those extra windows and concentrated on only one thing. While waiting for the compiler, I paid attention to the one thing I was working on, and "did I miss anything"? My net productivity went up, and it was much more relaxing. For some situations like being a Mom or a short-order cook, multi-tasking is unavoidable. For the rest of us, it can be fool's gold.

Mindfulness is relaxing during various daily activities like driving, walking, and eating. Continuous activities like walking, hiking, biking, paddling, etc., are more calming and enjoyable if you pay attention to your surroundings and your breathing, and are examples of "mindfulness in motion".

Yoga and Tai Chi are both also healthy examples of mindfulness in motion. I do about 15 minutes of yoga stretches every night, which is stress relieving in itself because we store tension in our muscles, which can get released by stretch or massage. But it is especially relaxing if I do it mindfully instead of while watching TV. I cobbled together my yoga routine from classes I took over the years, from videos by Lilias Folan (there are a lot of yoga videos on the internet) and from books. You can stick to a beginner program and still learn good stretches. Tai Chi is a bit harder to self-teach because the movements are linked together and can be intricate, unless you find a really good instructional DVD. City adult ed or rec centers often offer classes.

Meditation

Sitting meditation is the most powerful method of stress relief I have found. Think of a time when you have spontaneously relaxed completely and gotten lost in the moment, your thoughts fading away as you are looking out on something beautiful, like a sunset over the ocean or behind some spectacular mountains. Meditation helps you to be able to cultivate that kind of feeling.

The simplest way is paying attention to your breath. This is just an extension of mindfulness, because you are supposed to be paying attention to what you are doing, and when you are sitting there, the only thing you are doing is breathing. You can observe the rise and fall of your diaphragm, or feel the breath going in and out. When a thought intrudes, just observe it, don't try to suppress it or get caught up in it, and just return your attention the breath. Easier said than done, but if you can gradually get yourself to do it for longer periods of time, working up to maybe 20 minutes, it's relaxing and helps with mental "fitness".

Some people find following the breath tedious, although you can get past that and start to enjoy it if you are disciplined enough to stick with it, which is well worth it. An alternative is the use of a focus sound, word, or phrase (also called a mantra). This is something to bring your attention back to, which should be a pleasant attractive sound. Sorry that I don't have the reference for this, but I read somewhere that words ending with the "n" or "m" sound were shown to be more relaxing by looking at brain waves.

Dr. Herbert Benson wrote a book called <u>The Relaxation Response</u> and has been doing research on the health benefits of stress management for a long time. He coined the phrase "relaxation response" because it acts as the antidote to the "fight or flight response", releasing relaxation hormones instead of stress hormones. He suggested the word "one" as a focus word, to be said on each out-breath, drawing it out like "onnnnnnne". You can also use a short phrase like "I am at peace", with "I am" on the in-breath, "at peace" on the out, again drawing out the sounds.

Like with the breath, when thoughts intrude, just gently move your attention back to the focus sound. After a while it becomes effortless, like the focus is saying itself. It's kind of similar to when a fragment of a song gets stuck in your head, but in a positive way. Your brain gets fascinated with the sound and its normal restless activity quiets down. Your focus can be repeated once per breath, as noted in the examples above. For me it works a little better if it's twice per breath, once on the in breath and once on the out. That is something you can experiment with to see which way calms your busy brain down better.

In addition to its relaxation benefits, meditation is a great way to train the mind. Far from being under control, our minds can flit from topic to topic. The terms "monkey mind" and "puppy mind" have been used to describe this. "Puppy" is useful because we can think of trying to training a puppy to heel on its leash. The focus, whether breath or sound, is analogous to the leash. Whenever the mind tries to wander off, we give it a gentle tug on the leash to bring the attention back to the focus.

This can seem a frustrating exercise, because the mind just wanders off again. But meditation teachers emphasize that bringing the attention back is precisely what is valuable for mind training. I like to think of bringing the attention back as "one rep". So if you have to do it many times during a meditation session, rather than feeling frustration, pat yourself on the back for doing lots of reps of mental exercise.

Many people find it difficult to get going with meditation. The "puppy mind" just jumps around the whole time and it can be frustrating. This is another good candidate for Stephen Guise's "mini-habits" approach. Yoga teacher Lilias Folan recommends "minute vacations", or short meditation sessions of maybe a minute in length[135]. This could be introduced as one of your mini-habits, at a specific time or when you're feeling wound up. Just take a nice deep breath, close your eyes, and pay attention to your breath for a minute. Hopefully it will settle into more relaxing and deeper "belly breathing" rather than the more shallow chest breathing many of us do when stressed out. You could then slowly ramp this up by gradually increasing the length of your session over time and/or sneaking it in more than once during your day.

I do "mindfulness in motion" during biking, hiking, yoga, etc., and also try to do sitting meditation for about 30 minutes every day. I'm a lot more relaxed than I was before I took up these practices.

Meditation and mindfulness have also been found to have excellent health benefits, and there are mindfulness-based stress reduction classes that are covered by health insurance, pioneered by Dr. Jon Kabat-Zinn[73]. Good motivation and instruction for meditation are presented in Dr. Benson's updated 2009 edition of The Relaxation Response[208].

Similar to a mantra is an affirmation, like "I can do this" when you're in the middle of a challenging task. But rather than for meditation, this is very helpful for positive thinking. The great runner Deana Kastor describes how diligently doing this took her career to the next level plus made life more enjoyable in her inspiring book Let Your Mind Run[207].

Conclusion

So here's to all of us working the four pillars into our lives. Move more often throughout out the day, and find an enjoyable physical activity that we look forward to rather than being a chore. Eat healthy food until pleasantly full, without cravings. Give and receive social support from family, friends, and community. Manage stress through mindfulness, meditation in motion, and sitting meditation. And there are many ways to work all of these together, like a nice mindful hike with friends followed by a picnic lunch together.

I hope you have enjoyed this book and find it helpful. Please follow my continuing adventures on https://bionicoldguy.home.blog/.

Appendix- Miscellaneous Topics

Bicycle Gearing

Conventional bike gearing is calculated using the number of teeth on the chainring in the front divided by the number of teeth on the sprocket in the back. This, multiplied times your wheel size, gives the gear inches. This is an interesting number which dates back to the old "penny farthing" bikes with the huge front wheel. The gear inches is the size of the wheel on one of those high wheelers you'd have to have to be the equivalent to the gear you are in on your bike. The higher this number, the further you go with a single revolution, but the harder it is to pedal.

Here's an example: my highest gear on my hybrid is a 48 tooth chainring, with an 11 tooth gear on the cassette in the back. 48/11 is 4.36, so that's like having a wheel 4.36 times as big as my actual one. My wheel is 28", to the gear inches is 4.36 times 28 = 122. So I'd have to have a penny farthing with a 10 foot diameter wheel to be equivalent to that! I'd need a stepladder to get on it, if I had the nerve to ride it (unlikely)! This is the English system of gearing.

A similar European system is to calculate "meters of development". Multiply the ratio of teeth in front to teeth in back times pi times the wheel size in meters. This gives how far the bike will go with one turn of the cranks. For example, my wheel size is 28" or 0.71 meters, so the development of my highest gear is 4.36 times pi times 0.71 = 9.72 meters. So my bike will travel 9.72 meters, or 32 feet, with one turn of the cranks in that gear.

For internal hub gears there's an additional factor. You still divide the chainring teeth by the sprocket in back. But then you multiply by a gear ratio for the hub. For example the famous Sturmey-Archer 3 speed hub has ratios of 0.75 in first, 1 in second gear, and 1.33 in third gear. So if you have a 26" wheel, 44 teeth up front and 14 in back, and you're in 3rd gear, you get 44/14 times 1.33 times 26 = 109 for your gear inches.

On Interpreting Scientific Studies

Many places throughout this and other books on exercise or nutrition topics, you'll find scientific studies cited as evidence. When you chase down these references, they will often seem to indeed support what is claimed. But some studies offer higher quality proof than others, so here's some background on how to try to tell the difference when you interpret them. The scientific method, in a nutshell is:

1. Observe some data. Propose a hypothesis that explains it.
2. Collect some more data to validate the hypothesis. This may disprove it or suggest modifications to it.

So an important thing is the quality of the data in these steps. I'll hit the high notes about that to see how to tell the quality of a study.

In nutritional science, the most obvious data to start with is population data. For example, we'll see below under "current (or recent) healthy populations" that many populations around the world are healthy on their traditional lifestyles and diet, and become considerably less healthy when adopting a more modern diet and way of life. A hypothesis that something is healthier about the combination of lower animal product consumption, lower consumption of processed foods, and higher amount of physical activity, fits the data nicely.

It could be that it has nothing to do with the animal product or the exercise, it's just the processed food, or that it's just the exercise, etc., or that it really does require the combination of all three. Suppose we instead offered the simpler hypothesis that it's healthier to eat less animal products. The data clearly does not yet prove that, so we would need more. This is typical with population studies, that there are multiple factors that need to be teased apart by further evidence.

The gold standard nutritional study is an interventional study on humans, with a larger enough sample size. Suppose five people in group 1 ate more meat and their health got worse, five people in group 2, the control, did not eat more meat and their health stayed the same. That's not enough of a sample size to be statistically significant (prove that the difference is not just random). A sample size of 100 in each group would be more compelling.

Ideally the intervention would be double blind, where neither scientists nor the people being studied (the subjects) know who is getting the intervention. This prevents the placebo effect, caused by the patient's belief in the intervention. You can do double-blind with something like a supplement pill: group 1 would get the supplement, group 2 gets a "sugar pill". You can sometimes also do it for single ingredients, for example by baking them into a cake that is fed to the subjects.

It's a lot harder with diet or lifestyle changes. If you put group 1 on the Atkins diet and group 2 on Pritikin, that's pretty hard to fake, everybody knows which diet they're on.

Interventional studies on animals that have enough anatomical similarities to humans can offer clues but not proof. Here's an obvious example: If you feed foods with cholesterol to rabbits they will get heart disease, pretty quickly. Does that prove the same will happen it humans? No, because rabbits are 100% herbivores whose digestive system has no way of handling cholesterol.

I didn't make this example up, by the way, such experiments really were run on rabbits in the 1950s and people really did suggest it meant it proves the same thing would happen in humans. Nonsense. If you do the same experiments with dogs, you'd see no effect at all, because they are carnivores whose digestion handles cholesterol just fine. If you did it on rats, who are omnivores, and saw an effect, that would be more intriguing. But it still wouldn't be proof. Rats could just be missing something like an important liver enzyme that humans have, that is important for handling cholesterol. You'd need to reproduce the result with humans to prove anything.

Some interventional studies on humans can be done in a relatively short time. You can take a group of people and put them on two different diets and see who loses the most weight in 6 months. Ideally, this would be done in a setting where the scientists controlled the food, and made sure the subjects didn't have access to snacks. A metabolic ward study where the subjects stay at a facility is the best example, and such studies have been done, but are quite expensive.

Instead, often two groups are given instructions to follow a diet, and then periodically interviewed to ask what they ate. This is obviously a lot lower quality than a ward study because people will vary on how well they comply with the diets (and possibly how honestly they answer the questions), but often this is the type of study done because it is easier. Some studies are much longer term. If you want to see the effect of an intervention on a chronic disease like heart disease it can take years. If you want to see the effects of an intervention on longevity it takes decades, so that type of study rarely if ever happens.

Probably the next best thing to an intervention study is a longitudinal study, where a significant number of people are followed for a long period of time. Measurements like blood cholesterol, triglycerides, etc. are periodically rechecked, and the people are periodically interviewed about what they are eating, smoking habits, exercise levels, etc. This goes on for many years and you follow their longevity as well as risks of developing various diseases.

An example is the Adventist Health Study[114]. Now you have to do statistical analysis to try to get clues or trends. When you have multiple similar studies you can do a statistical on all of them called a meta-analysis. If properly done this is more compelling than the results of any single study.

The statistics needs to be interpreted carefully. For example, you might find that "people who drank more coffee had a higher risk of lung cancer". Can we conclude coffee causes lung cancer? This is a classic example of "correlation is not causation". It turns out heavy smokers often have a caffeine habit as well as a nicotine habit. Smoking caused the lung cancer, but coffee drinking accidentally correlated with it.

On the other hand, if coffee had correlated negatively with lung cancer, that would make it unlikely that coffee caused lung cancer. This is because of step 1 of the scientific method: The hypothesis that coffee causes lung cancer does not fit the data.

An example is a hypothesis about legumes. Legumes contain phytic acid, which is called an "antinutrient" because it interferes with the body absorbing other nutrients. So we could hypothesize "legumes contain phytic acid, an antinutrient, so legumes will lead to a poorer health". But there are data from populations around the world showing the opposite. For example, it turns out that elderly people who consume the most legumes live the longest. It is a very strong correlation, more than any other variable looked at[22]. Also, other studies have shown that legumes correlate with reduced disease risk. Our hypothesis does not fit either of these pieces of information, so it is unlikely.

Another important thing to check when looking at a study is who funded the study. In the US, if the funding is from the National Institutes of Health, there are no strings attached. But if the funding is from an industry group, such as the American Beverage Association, the results of the study are more suspect. Statistics have shown that authors of a study are much more likely to come up with results that are favorable to sources of funding like that. It's not necessarily lack of integrity on the scientists' part, the funding source could just introduce an unconscious bias.

Funding comes up in another way. In his book <u>Low Fat Lies, High Fat Fraud</u>, Dr. Kevin Vigilante describes how back in the 90s he tried to get a grant for a study on the health benefits of the Mediteranean diet. But his proposal was rejected with essentially the explanation "everybody knows the healthiest way to eat is high carb/low fat. We don't need to investigate alternatives".

This is an example of a need for a "paradigm shift". When the majority of scientists believe a theory, it can be hard to get evidence accepted if it contradicts the theory. Only when multiple studies, confirmed in by multiple research teams, coming at the problem from different angles, does the "herd" finally shift. In the case of the theory that high carb/low fat is healthy, it took evidence accumulating over years to cause this shift: "Here's this study that shows better results on a higher fat lower carb diet. And here's some evidence that there are good carbs and bad carbs, and here's other evidence that there are good fats and bad fats, and if we do a meta-analysis of all these studies it turns out the correlation between dietary fat intake and heart disease is weaker than previously thought", etc.

Physical Activity, Health, and Longevity

A sedentary lifestyle is a major risk factor for conditions like heart disease, type II diabetes and arthritis. Most adults are not meeting minimum exercise guidelines, and activity levels decrease with age, so our health care and long-term care systems are very overburdened due to largely preventable diseases. And while the problem of our growing number of overweight and obese Americans (and now people around the world) is caused to a certain extent by bad (and supersized) diet, the other major contributor is inactivity.

Recently it has been recognized that many of what are normally thought of as effects of aging are in fact largely attributable to inactivity[26,141,142,147]. The biology of why staying active prevents the body's "decay" is explained in <u>Younger Next Year</u>[21], and lots of books detail the health benefits of exercise, see for example <u>Fitness and Health</u>[141]. It's been clearly demonstrated that exercise adds life to your years as well as years to your life. To me the "adding life to your years" is the most important: It can be the difference between being vibrant right up to the end of life, or suffering a long debilitating decline.

Various measures of "fitness", including cardiovascular fitness, muscle strength, and flexibility, diminish relentlessly with age in sedentary adults. Eventually this leads to the "frailty" of older adults: when your fitness has declined enough, you are no longer "functionally fit" to perform everyday tasks. You may not have the flexibility to reach the upper cabinets in the kitchen or tie your own shoes, or the strength to pick up a child or a bag of groceries, and may get winded just going up a flight of stairs. And your walking gait may turn into a shuffle as you get progressively stiffer and weaker.

These are things we normally think of as occurring in much older people, but a national study of 10,000 women aged 40-55 showed the scary result that more than 25% already had difficulty with everyday activities[110]. Due to loss of muscle mass, your metabolism will relentlessly slow down and your body fat percentage will creep up, causing your weight to increase even if the amount of food you eat remains constant, known as the dreaded "middle age spread".

Dieting without exercising only makes the problem worse: it can lead to more loss of muscle mass, a slower metabolism, and the weight quickly coming back. Lack of weight-bearing exercise means insufficient stimulus for bone tissue growth, which contributes to osteoporosis. Your mobility may also be severely hampered by conditions like arthritis which are made worse by inactivity. Since it hurts to move, a vicious cycle of moving even less may result. Obviously, all of this is getting into serious reduction in quality of life. Eventually the frailty can lead to an inability to take care of yourself, and possibly ending up in a nursing home.

Use it or Lose It

Loss of muscle mass (sarcopenia) is one of many aspects that's often thought of as an "inevitable" aspect of aging, as is gradually diminished aerobic capacity, muscle and bone loss, and gradual increase in blood pressure. But all of these can be improved dramatically by staying active[44,117]: it's use it or lose it.

The main areas where lack of physical activity causes us to "lose it" are aerobic capacity and strength. Aerobic capacity declines when we simply don't move around enough. Getting the equivalent of walking a couple of miles a day from activities of daily living is probably a bare minimum.

Higher end activity is also important: the ability to exercise at least for short periods at higher MET levels is a strong predictor of longevity. A "metabolic equivalent" or MET of 1 is how much energy you're using sitting in a recliner. Good longevity is predicted for those who can exercise at a level that uses at least 8 times that much (or 8 METs, equivalent to running or brisk cycling) compared to people who can only achieve a more moderate level of 5 Mets[3]. Higher intensity exercise in the form of interval training also improves arterial flexibility[58], lowering risk for stroke and heart attack.

So exercising at a higher level for short periods at least a couple of times a week is a good idea. For those who don't like formal exercise programs, climbing stairs is a good activity of daily living for higher intensity. Climbing a few flights briskly a couple of times a week would be a good start. You can turn stair climbing into interval training also, as I showed in chapter 3.

The last area is strength. There's the famous "Wolfe's law" in biology which states that bones will adapt to the loads that are placed upon them[198], but a similar thing happens for muscles and other important tissues in the body. It's also true in nature as shown in the photo.

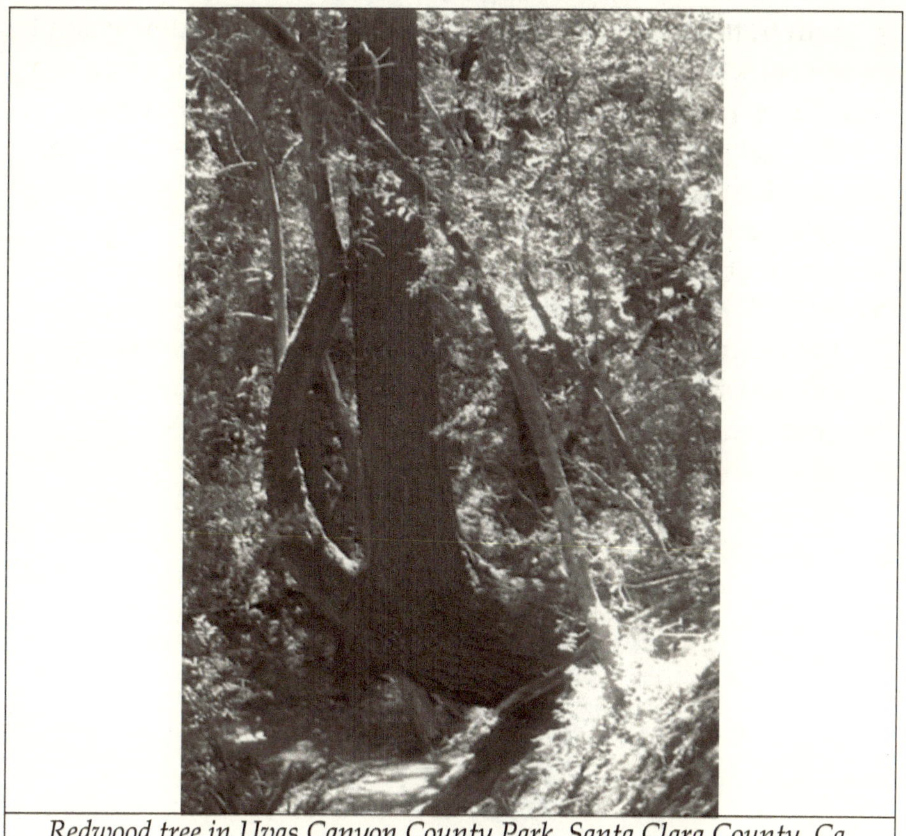

Redwood tree in Uvas Canyon County Park, Santa Clara County, Ca.

A living organism will respond to the loading on it to make an optimal structure by growing new tissue where needed (wood growth in the case of a tree). This redwood grew sideways out of the bank decades ago, then turned up to strive for more light. This puts a lot of bending stress at the base, so it grew enormously thick there. Conversely, if you are never applying any load, the body assumes you don't need strong bones or muscles and will tend to recycle those cells. One of the scariest statistics of aging is that if we are not active we can lose 3 to 5% of our muscle mass every decade as we age (www.health.harvard.edu/staying-healthy/preserve-your-muscle-mass). If that statistic doesn't frighten you, perhaps this picture is worth a thousand words:

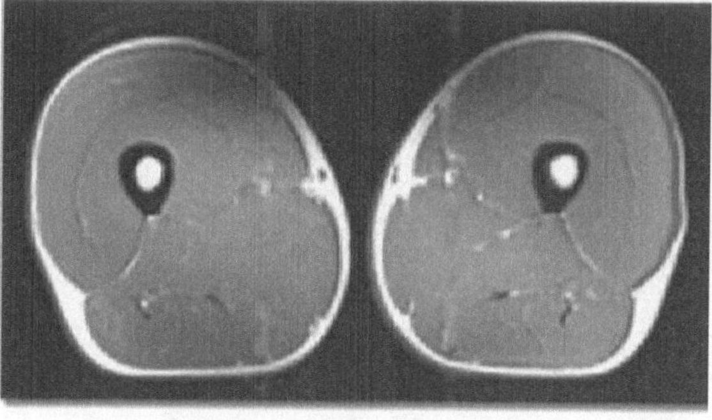

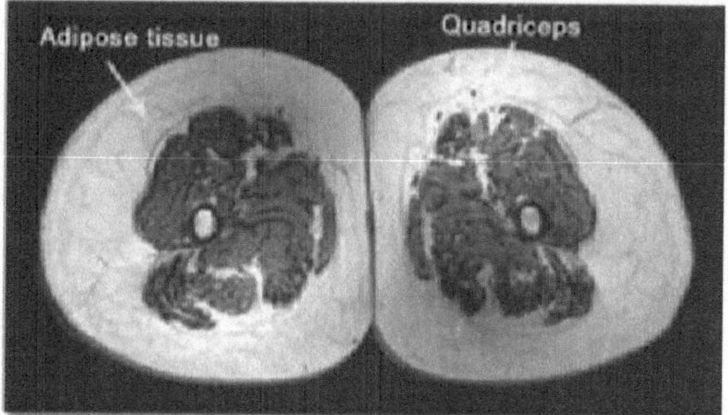

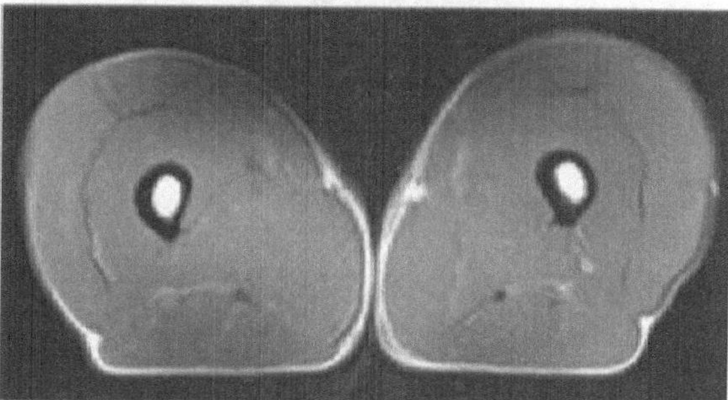

From Cycling and triathlon coach Joe Friel's Blog (www.joefrielsblog.com/2013/09)

Fighting off losing muscle mass as we age. These are scans of the cross-sections of men's left and right thigh muscles. For the 40 year old and 70 year old triathletes, the thin white ring around the outside is fat, the small black circle surrounding the white circle in the middle is the thigh bone (femur), and the rest is muscle.

For the 74 Year old sedentary man the large white outside is now fat. Even the femur is smaller so he's lost bone as well as a lot of muscle

This is a single anecdotal result, but a recent controlled study confirmed it for a group of serious masters cyclists aged 55-79 who averaged over 100 miles per week. There was no significant age-related loss in the quad muscles with age[215]. This contrasted sharply with a sedentary control group of similar age range. Immune system function in the masters cyclists was also significantly superior to that of the control group[216].

Don't sit too much

Sitting for too long is a risk factor even for those who have an exercise routine. Sitting too much leads to a higher risk of death from all causes[154], a higher likelihood of disability in activities of daily living[30], and higher risk of cardiac and metabolic issues[59].

The Anti-aging and Metabolic Benefits of Resistance Training and HIIT

As we've seen, there are multiple health and anti-aging benefits of exercise. Accumulating research is showing strong evidence that these results are even better for resistance training and higher intensity cardio (HIIT). There is a good discussion of this in Jonathan Bailor's <u>The Calorie Myth</u>. There is also a nice overview of the literature in Ref. 221.

Resistance training has a dramatic effect on muscle, both by reversing sarcopenia (muscle loss), and improving mitochondrial activity (the mitochondria are the energy powerhouses in our cells, especially important in muscles)[222, 223, 229]. HIIT is more effective than lower intensity cardio to lower insulin resistance[225], reduce metabolic syndrome[224], and reduce dangerous visceral fat[226], and improve cardiovascular risk factors[228]. All of these will have a dramatic positive effect on the metabolism and are an important adjunct to the dietary "reset" discussed in chapter 4.

Gut Microbiome

Our gut microbiome consists of about 100 trillion bacteria in our intestines, ten times the number of cells in the human body. This has a huge effect on health and is affected by the foods we eat- way beyond eating yogurt. Here are some examples of the health effects.

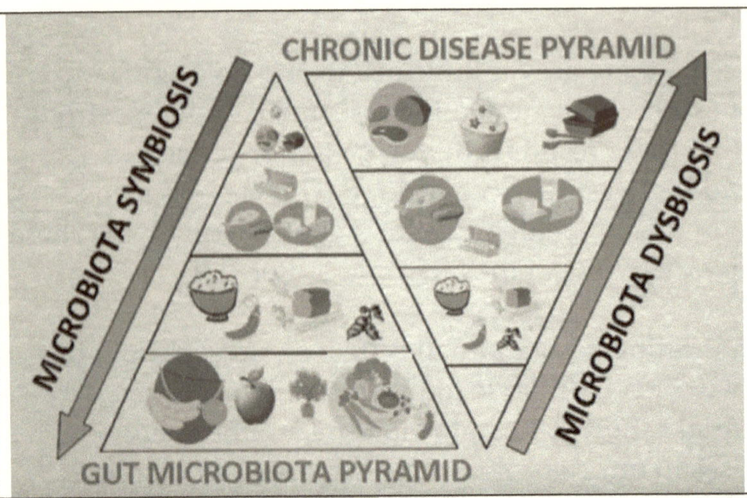

Effects of different foods on good bacteria and bad bacteria in the gut. Vegetable, fruits, legumes, minimally processed grains, and beans nourish good bacteria while junk food, and excess meats, fish, eggs, and dairy nourish the bad bacteria[152]. I'm assuming this result is for people whose digestive systems handle grains and legumes well.

A recent paper suggest that refined carbs cause a change in gut bacteria that leads to an inflammatory response, which the author suggests is a primary cause of obesity[180]. For some of us this problem may be enough to cause obesity, for others it may be milder but still a major cause of cravings.

The choline in animal products (meat, eggs, dairy), and the L-carnitine in red meat, acted on by our gut flora, produce the toxic compound TMAO, which raises the risk of heart failure, kidney failure, atherosclerosis[150,11,101], and cancer[2].

The gut microbiome is readily modifiable by changing our diet. Eating a vegetarian diet changes the gut flora over time so that the bacteria that produce TMAO are no longer present[43]. In a single month of eating a vegetarian diet, there's also a major shift in general towards good bacteria and away from bad bacteria. This reduces intestinal inflammation dramatically, which results in improved metabolic and immunological factors in patients with metabolic diseases[78]. Diets high in phytate (in grains and legumes) modify the gut flora so it is better able to aid in digesting phytates[93]. High fiber content from plant foods also promotes bacteria that produce beneficial short chain fatty acids[151].

Protein: Recommended Amount and Safe Upper Limit

The recommended daily allowance of protein is 0.18 grams per Kg of ideal body weight (0.4 grams per pound). If you're currently overweight, your ideal weight is what you'd like to get down to. Physically active individuals need more, so multiply this by about 2 for serious strength trainers (who need protein to repair and build muscle), and by about 1.5 for endurance athletes (who also need to repair muscle, and actually burn a little protein during longer sessions)[4]. I'm not sure what the recommendation is for non-athletes who just participate in some strength training or cardio to stay in shape, probably a factor of safety of 1.5 is fine.

There is concern that long term consumption of excess protein in adulthood, especially from animal sources, raises cancer risks and all-cause mortality[146]. But an interesting recent finding is that bumping up protein a bit after age 65 helps to ward off muscle loss and frailty. Also protein consumption correlates with higher serum levels of insulin-like growth factor 1 (igf-1) which in excess increases risk for mortality. But after 65 people tend to be deficient in igf-1, another benefit to increasing protein intake after age 65[88]. But the recommended amount after 65 is still not too high, like around 0.27 grams per kg of bodyweight (0.6 grams per pound). Protein should also be higher for children and young adults who are still growing, so maybe the number for strength trainers should be used for them (0.36 grams per Kg or 0.8 grams per pound). Excess Igf-1 is not a concern while still growing.

Recommended Daily Amount of Protein			
	Sedentary	Moderately Active or endurance athlete	Strength athlete
Adults	0.4 grams/lb. of lean bodyweight	0.6 grams/lb. of ideal bodyweight	0.8 grams/lb. of ideal bodyweight
Seniors 65+	0.6 grams/lb. of ideal bodyweight	0.6 grams/lb. of ideal bodyweight	0.8 grams/lb. of ideal bodyweight

Some diets, such as the high meat version of the paleo diet, advocate higher consumption of protein than the RDA. It is controversial whether that is a good idea long term because of the longevity issues. But even in the short term, it is important from a health perspective to know the safe upper limit for protein. As part of metabolizing protein, your liver has to convert nitrogen in the blood to urea. Exceeding the upper limit the liver can handle can lead to various symptoms of protein toxicity. Your kidneys have to handle the urea load from the digestion of proteins, so excess protein can impair kidney function.

The theoretical safe upper limit to avoid protein toxicity is 3.5-4.6 grams per Kg of body weight (1.6-2.1 grams per pound of body weight. Throwing a bit of safety factor in, a recommended upper limit is 2 to 2.5 grams per Kg of body weight (0.9-1.1 grams per pound of body weight)[4]. There may be mitigating factors from other aspects of the diet, for example excess protein can lead to excess acid in the blood that needs to be cleared by the kidneys, called potential renal acid load, or PRAL[131]. Eating lots of greens reduces PRAL and may offset this. Authors who believe in higher protein diets or higher meat consumption tend to push it closer to the safe upper limit, and are counting on these mitigating factors.

Can Vegans Get Enough Protein?

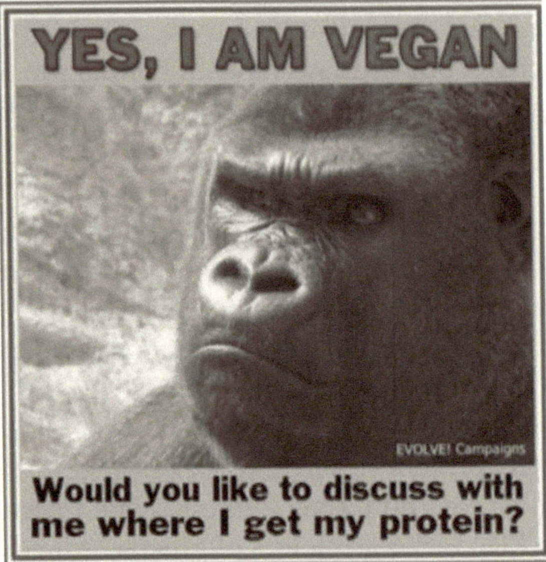

[https://happyherbivore.com/2010/12/vegan-paleo/]

This is a question vegans get so tired of answering that I've seen the picture above on T-shirts. There are two main issues: does plant food provide complete protein (a balanced set of amino acids), and does plant food have enough protein density so you can get your daily requirement from eating a reasonable amount of calories?

It's been known that the answers to both of these is yes since as early as 1971, when Frances Moore Lappe's book <u>Diet for a Small Planet</u> came out. So I was disappointed to see these same old issues raised in Dr. Mark Hyman's recent book <u>Food: What the Heck Should I Eat</u>? I should note that Dr. Hyman actually advocates eating a reduced amount of meat, which he recommends using as a condiment (he uses the term "condi-meat"). It is only his contention that plant-based sources of protein are inadequate that I disagree with.

Plant Protein Completeness:

There are 9 amino acids that the body cannot produce (therefore called essential), that we need to get from protein in food. Animal products tend to have a good amount of each of these, so are considered "complete". Plant sources tend to be deficient in one or more, but by eating a combination of sources as suggested in healthy vegan or wfpb diets, we are assured of a complete supply[97].

Back when Ms. Lappe wrote her book, it was thought you had to do the combining at each meal, and she gave instructions on how to do so. She also pointed out that traditional populations that could not afford a lot of animal products have all come up with solutions for this in their diets, for example rice and tofu, or tortillas and beans. But it is now known that our bodies are smart enough to do the combining throughout the day, as long as a variety of plant foods is eaten[97].

It is also claimed that meat is a better source of the amino acid leucine than plant sources[71], but there is actually concern that excess consumption of leucine from meat sources contributes to type II diabetes, cancer and aging[99, 159].

Getting Enough Protein From Plants:

Here is where Dr. Hyman got the math wrong. He cites this example: 100 grams of beef has 36 grams of protein, while 100 grams of tofu has 9 grams of protein. So this seems like you need to eat a lot more tofu to get your protein. But that amount of beef is 217 calories, while that amount of tofu is 70 calories. To get the same amount of protein as you get from beef, you'd need to eat 400 grams of tofu, but that is only 280 calories, not so much more than the beef. There are even denser sources of protein. White button mushrooms have 3.6 g protein/100g but only 23.8 calories, so 36 grams of protein is 238 calories[169]. Nutritional yeast has 9 grams of protein for a 60 calorie serving.

There is also a surprising amount of protein in vegetables[170], for example: 1 avocado has 10 grams, 1 cup broccoli - 5 grams, 1 cup spinach - 5 grams, 2 cups cooked kale - 5 grams, 1 cup cooked sweet potato – 5 grams.

Although I believe you can get enough protein from plant foods, it helps to be knowledgeable about the concentrated sources like tofu, tempeh, and seitan (which was traditionally called Fu in Japan). Some authors say don't worry about protein, just eat a variety of plant foods and you'll get plenty. I think that may be going too far. Some traditional people that are quite healthy on a near-vegan diet are short of stature, but it is not genetic. An example is the members of the Pima tribe in Mexico still eating their traditional diet and those in Arizona eating closer to the SAD. As discussed in chapter 4, those on the traditional diet are much healthier, but those on the modern diet are taller[181].

The moral is not to switch to the modern diet or that you can't get enough protein without meat, but you need to audit your diet to see assure that you're really getting adequate protein (like the recommend daily allowance discussed above), and maybe add concentrated sources if necessary. As I discuss under meat alternatives below, for those like me that are not good cooks, there are some healthy brands of meat alternatives like Turkey and Sweet Earth. Just chop them up and throw them in stirfry or salad and you have a delicious meal with plenty of protein. There are also good plant-based supplements in powder form.

I can't resist throwing in this about nutritional yeast: A favorite Sci Fi author of mine was Dr. Isaac Asimov. He wrote a great novel, <u>The Caves of Steel</u>, in 1953 that was both sci-fi and a detective story involving a human cop partnered with a robot. It depicted a future society short on resources where protein needs were met by growing vast quantities of yeast.

Health and Longevity Aspects of Some Controversial Foods

Food and Inflammation

Inflammation is mentioned in discussing various foods below, so I'll review it first here. Chronic inflammation is considered an important risk factor for various diseases. It also is a major contributor to the aging process, in fact the medical term "Inflamm-aging" has been coined[206]. So it's important to have an anti-inflammatory diet, containing more foods that have an anti-inflammatory effect (like fruits and veggies) and fewer with a pro-inflammatory effect. Anti-inflammatory foods also reduce inflammation and delayed-onset muscle soreness after exercise, without interfering with beneficial effects of recovery[6].

Good and Bad fats

Fat is an important nutrient. It's unfortunate we don't any better word for it because even the name can bring up negative images, like bacon grease congealed in a pan. Yuck! We also use the same word for fat in food and fat around our midsections, another negative association. We went through a low fat era and it has left many people fat phobic. To this day I have to catch myself reading an author who proposes low-carb/high-fat: "More than 50% fat. Are you crazy? OK, calm down, he says it's healthy fat, let's hear what he has to say".

There are good and bad fats, and you can eat a decent amount of good fat and still be healthy and lean. To understand good and bad, it helps to know how heart disease actually happens, which is discussed below under "Saturated Fat". And bad fats contribute to chronic inflammation, which we've already seen is bad.

Trans-fats: <u>very bad</u>. There is overall consensus that trans-fats should be avoided like the plague. Some authors call them the ugly fat. They promote inflammation, heart disease, and other diseases. The main source of trans fats in the diet is hydrogenated vegetable oil, found in processed foods and my grandma's tub of Crisco.

In the US we've finally gotten around to labeling trans fats, so you should look for 0 grams. But it can still be misleading, manufacturers are allowed to round it off to zero if it's less than 1 gram per serving. Cool Whip has 0 g trans fats for a serving size of two tablespoons, but *who uses two tablespoons*? You use a great big pile of it. If it's really 0.9 grams per two tablespoons, and they rounded down to 0, and you're using a cup of it (16 tablespoons) you'd really be getting 7.2 grams of trans-fats (2 grams is considered the healthy upper limit per day).

If you do use processed food, avoid anything that has hydrogenated in the label. But trans fats also occur from the high heats used to process commercial vegetable oils which is why expeller pressed oils are recommended instead, and they can occur from cooking unsaturated oils (especially polyunsaturated) at too high of a temperature[145].

What is not often mentioned is that if you avoid commercial oils, cooking oils at high temperature, and processed food with "hydrogenated" ingredients, the major remaining source of trans-fats is those that occur naturally in animal foods[41], which have been shown to have similar bad health effects to those in hydrogenated vegetable oils[10].

Omega3 and Omega6 Polyunsaturated Fats: Vegetable oils are polyunsaturated, and there is also polyunsaturated fat in animal products. Polyunsaturated fats contain omega3 and omega6 fatty acids. Too high of a ratio of omega6 to omega3 in your diet is inflammatory, leading to many health issues including heart disease and arthritis[118]. The ideal proportion is around 1:1, while when eating SAD we may be closer to 20:1. Most vegetable oils have a high ratio, the exception is canola which is 2:1 (canola is controversial as discussed below). Fatty fish are high in omega3 as long as they are wild and not farmed[71], and so are walnuts and flax and chia seeds (you have to grind the seeds before eating so your body absorbs the omega3).

Omega3 is why there is a recommendation to eat fish oil. Because of concerns over mercury and other pollutants, it is good idea to find a source that has been molecularly distilled or independently tested not to have pollutants[71]. In the US we have "USP certified", and there are quality mail order varieties like Nordic Naturals.

There is a whole other discussion about the benefits of fatty acids like ALA, DHA, and EPA[71] (types of omega3) and their health benefits. Plant sources like walnuts and flax do not provide DHA or EPA, just ALA, and your body will convert the ALA to DHA and EPA, but inefficiently. So there is some concern over getting enough DHA and EPA if you are vegan or following a wfpb diet with a low amount of animal foods. This can be addressed by taking supplements sourced from algae[79].

Dairy and beef both contain unsaturated fats as well as saturated. If they are from grass fed animals they contain a higher percentage of omega3 fatty acids compared to commercial grain fed products, which are high in omega6, which is the reason for the recommendation to eat grass-fed. Monounsaturated Fats are present in large percentage in olive oil, nuts, avocados, and canola oil, and other vegetable oils labeled "high-oleic". Oleic acid is an omega9 fatty acid, and is considered to be generally beneficial[134].

Monounsaturated Fats are present in large percentage in olive oil, nuts, avocados, and canola oil, and other vegetable oils labeled "high-oleic". Oleic acid is an omega9 fatty acid, and is considered to be generally beneficial[134]. Monounsaturated fats have healthy properties including decreased risk for breast cancer (especially if the monounsaturated fat replaces polyunsaturated fat in the diet[164]), and improved glycemic control in diabetics[28].

Fats and Endothelial Function

Arteries are capable of expanding (dilating) in response to blood flow, triggered by healthy functioning of their inner layer, the endothelium. Not only are they flexible but they are active tissue that responds to nitric oxide released by the endothelium by expanding. This response is called flow-mediated (vaso)dilation, or FMD. Consumption of a high fat meal significantly impairs FMD for several hours[156]. This happens whether it is saturated fat or vegetable oils, including extra virgin olive oil. This effect does not happen for evoo combined with vegetables at a mea[136], or if vinegar, especially red wine or balsamic vinegar, is consumed along with the evoo[133]. The vinegar effect can also be replicated by just eating red grapes[15].

Degraded endothelial function is a symptom of coronary artery disease (CAD)[20]. I have not seen proof that the short-term impairment of endothelial function after a meal leads over time to chronic impairment, which could result in CAD. But most authors seem to assume that is does, which may be because high fat consumption also raises markers of inflammation and oxidative stress in the same time period the arterial stiffening is occurring. The markers are not raised if the fat is from a whole plant-food source like avocados or whole olives[77].

It is suspected that the rich amount of healthy phytochemicals in the whole plant food cancels out any negative effect of the fat. I haven't found references that the combination of saturated fats and plant foods blunts the effect on FMD also, but it seems logical that it would. So veggies sauteed in butter would have saturated fat but might have a more benign effect on FMD than a hamburger by itself.

The effect of fat on FMD is one reason why some wfpb proponents like Dr. Caldwell Esselstyn advise minimizing consumption of all fats including added oil. Dr. Esselstyn treats patients with advanced CAD, many who suffer from angina. In their case, impaired FMD after a meal could trigger an angina attack and should clearly be avoided. For the rest of us, it might be ok to loosen up from "no oil" to "oil in moderation", especially if we make sure to consume veggies or vinegar with the oil.

Saturated Fat

The link between saturated fat and atherothrombosis, the main danger in coronary artery disease, is not as clear cut as previously thought. However, as we'll see, saturated fat also plays a role in other conditions.

Saturated Fat and Coronary Artery Disease

Coronary artery disease is caused by the formation and progression of coronary plaques (atherosclerosis). Plaques can be stable, and act like a "partially clogged pipe", which can cause angina. Arteries are not really pipes, they are active flexible tubes, as we just saw under flow-mediated vasodilation, so it's really more like "partially clogged flexible tube". But in any case the most dangerous plaques are unstable plaques, which account for the vast majority of heart attacks[42] when they rupture. The mechanism is like a pimple bursting, leading to a severe inflammatory response and possible complete blockage of an artery.

Increases in saturated fat in the diet are well known to correlate with increases in ldl in the blood[17] and since ldl was felt to be a primary risk factor for coronary artery disease, this put blame on saturated fat. However, recent evidence shows it is more complicated. It appears that the key step in the initiation of plaque formation (stable or unstable) is the penetration of the arterial wall (the endothelium), and the greatest risk factor for that is ldl particle number: if you have high ldl but the ldl particles are all large (sometimes colloquially called fluffy), the ldl particle number will be low.

But if they are the smaller dangerous kind, the particle number, or ldl-p, will be high. The reason why it is small dense ldl that is dangerous is that penetration of the endothelium is actually caused by oxidized ldl[84], and small dense ldl is more likely to oxidize. When you get your cholesterol measured it is ldl-c. There is a test using nuclear magnetic resonance for ldl-p but it is not usually ordered by doctors (or paid for by insurance). However, a high ratio of hdl to triglycerides correlates with larger ldl, so your ldl is likely to be benign if you have high hdl relative to triglycerides. This can happen for a diet high in saturated fat but low in carbs, especially refined carbs[63].

This would let saturated fat off the hook for heart disease. However, the combination of saturated fat and refined carbs could still be dangerous (for one thing it is known to be highly inflammatory)[112], and should be avoided. That should not be a problem if you eat a diet that minimizes refined carbs.

Even with this new evidence, there is also strong evidence that if you keep refined carbs low, and keep ldl very low (less than 70), it will not lead to coronary plaque[113]. So proponents of diets like wfpb, that still recommend keeping saturated fats low, are basing it on this cholesterol goal. They argue that the poor results for "normal" blood numbers mean that the standards are not strict enough.

It's quite possible that both approaches are right. You can keep hdl high and triglycerides low by avoiding refined carbs, and eating plenty of good fat which drives up hdl, and not worry about saturated fat. Or you can keep ldl and triglycerides very low. Or you can do both ("belt and suspenders") by following a version of wfpb which has reduced saturated fat but emphasizes more of the healthy fats like omega3 and monounsaturated discussed above.

There is one puzzling piece of data that does not fit the high hdl/triglycerides argument: An African population, the Masai, do get fairly severe plaque in their coronary arteries, but it appears to be stable (discussed below under "Rural Africans"), on a traditional diet high in saturated fat and low in carbohydrates which does not contain processed foods. If there is a mechanism by which saturated fat, in the absence of refined carbs, could lead to stable plaque, it could still be dangerous because there are other conditions (like dementia, renal failure, erectile dysfunction, and angina) in which arterial plaque formation is implicated even if it is stable.

Upon searching the literature, I was able to find only one potential mechanism: It is possible to ingest oxidized cholesterol directly from animal products, which could cause plaque formation[106,32]. This still appears to exonerate saturated fat for plaque formation, but implicates at least some animal foods.

Saturated Fat and Other Diseases

Ingestion of excess saturated fat contributes to lipotoxicity, a metabolic syndrome that may be involved in "several inflammatory pathways, contributing to disease progression in chronic inflammation, autoimmunity, allergy, cancer, atherosclerosis, hypertension, and heart hypertrophy as well as other metabolic and degenerative diseases" [38,76].
Dietary saturated fat correlates negatively with binding of insulin-like growth factor-1 (igf-1) which contributes to cancer risk[64,160]. However, this was found in population-based studies and it is not clear whether the participants were also consuming refined carbohydrates. We already know that combination is bad, so this is not necessarily evidence that saturated fat alone is a cancer risk factor.

Ldl is positively correlated with calcification of heart valves[123]. Not enough is known at this point, it may be that it is ldl particle number that really matters, not ldl, as seems to be the case for atherosclerosis. But the mechanism must differ at least somewhat with that for atherosclerosis, because valve calcification does not respond to statin therapy[89].

This seems to be an overlooked area for research. In the US about 80,000 to 85,000 heart valve replacements are done per year[204]. At least half of these probably involve using tissue valves as replacements, so there are 40,000 or so of those a year. You'd have to track the recipients down and follow them in a longitudinal study, occasionally auditing their diet, and monitor how quickly their new valves calcify. I'm officially volunteering for such a study.

In the meantime, because not enough is known at this point, I've decided to be conservative and stay low on saturated fat, since I have a replacement tissue valve that I'd like to maximize the life of. So, sadly, butter is not back for me, except as a special treat.

Controversial Fats

Olives are undoubtedly healthy, but olive oil is still a processed food, although in its extra-virgin form (or "evoo"), it is one of the least processed plant oils. It can contain up to 20% saturated fat. If you're concerned about that you can find varieties with as low as 7½%. Many nutritionists consider evoo healthy, especially because of its monounsaturated fat content, and it is a well-known part of the Mediterranean diet.

Others, like many wfpb authors, consider it unhealthy (though maybe "less bad" than other sources of fat like animal products or other vegetable oils). They are also concerned about the misconception about the Mediterranean diet that it makes food more "heart healthy" if you pour olive oil on it (like sopping bread in it as you'll see people do at restaurants).

I grant them that point. But if you want to claim that all oils are unhealthy and you should eat all of them in moderation, I'd argue that evoo is among the "least unhealthy". If you want to use a bit of oil as a yellow food to get you to eat more green foods, evoo is a good choice. It's what I put in my refillable oil sprayer to sauté veggies.

Coconut oil is predominantly saturated fat, but also contains some medium chain triglycerides (MCTs) which have beneficial properties. It is often claimed to be a healthy oil. High consumption of unprocessed coconuts appears to be healthy for Pacific Island populations like the Tokeluans[125] and Kitavans[85], but I don't know of studies proving this to be true for coconut oil, a processed food from coconuts.

As for the MCTs, coconut oil actually contains a small percentage of these. It does contain a large amount of lauric acid, a medium chain fatty acid, but that is not the same as a medium chain triglyceride. A review of how it is metabolized concluded: "It is therefore inaccurate to consider coconut oil to contain either predominantly medium-chain fatty acids or predominantly medium-chain triglycerides. Thus, the evidence on medium-chain triglycerides cannot be extrapolated to coconut oil"[182].

Other than the relatively high saturated fat content for a plant oil, I have not seen evidence for coconut oil being particularly unhealthy either. Its status appears to depend on the science concerning saturated fat (above).

Canola oil is a vegetable oil made from the rapeseed plant, which contains erucic acid (with deleterious health effects). Canola was developed by hybridizing (through cross-breeding) the rapeseed plant to obtain a much lower erucic content (about 4% of that of rapeseed oil), and the name canola is short for "Canadian oil low acid". This is the only vegetable oil with a good ratio of omega6 to omega3 (a 2:1 ratio).

This oil is controversial. Many people rail against it, making it seem like a frankenfood. One reason is the erucic acid content, but it has been specifically bred to minimize that. The other reasons given to avoid it are the same reasons to avoid any commercially processed oil, so I don't get why canola is singled out. If you use organic, expeller pressed oil, it is not genetically modified, nor has it undergone any high temperature processing or deodorization, nor will it contain trans fats

I have not seen any reasons given why the organic, expeller pressed form of canola is bad for you. A final note on canola oil is that there was a significant amount of it used in the Mediterranean-style diet in the Lyons heart study[183], which showed drastically reduced heart disease risk compared to the control group on a diet similar to the SAD. Not bad for a frankenfood.

Animal Foods

The discussion in this section is about excess consumption of animal foods. As seen below under "Current (or Recent) Healthy Populations", there are populations known to have good health and longevity that get up to 15% of their calories from animal products. How far above that is the line for "excess" is a controversial point.

A main concern in the past about animal foods (except fish) has been saturated fat intake. We've discussed the saturated fat and heart disease connection, which is less clear than previously thought. If you are still concerned about saturated fat, you can go with leaner choices of animal foods.

Paleo authors[19] and others like Dr. Mark Hyman[71] suggest healthy options for animal foods (grass-fed beef, eggs from pasture-raised chickens, etc.), which improves their omega3 content, among other benefits. I agree this is a good idea. What I don't know to what extent it mitigates the negative health aspects about to be discussed.

All animal foods (dairy, meat, eggs, and fish) have some negative effects on gut bacteria, which as discussed above has important health effects[152]. For example, they can cause the gut bacteria to produce the toxic compound TMAO, which has various disease risks. They are also implicated in inflammatory bowel disease because "Diets rich in animal protein and animal fat cause a decrease in beneficial bacteria in the intestine"[16]. Replacing some of the protein in the diet from animal foods with plant-based protein is associated with significantly lower all-cause mortality[146]. A final concern is that animal foods contain naturally occurring trans fats[41].

Dairy

Both wfpb and paleo advocates consider dairy to be an unhealthy food. It is inflammatory, and there are other health issues with dairy in the nonfat portion of it (such as skim milk). Ironically, despite it being touted as good for the bones, increased dairy consumption correlates with higher rates of bone fractures and osteoporosis[104]. Dairy is also a significant source of estrogen, associated with acne and male infertility[72], and increased cancer risk[100].

I quoted the statistic above the Americans are eating 7 times as much cheese as 100 years ago. This is also triple the amount we were eating in the early 1970s[108]. Processed foods are a significant hidden source of cheese, so if you avoid them you will automatically reduce your cheese consumption as a side effect.

Meat

Many authors argue that meat is now ok because the saturated fat picture is not as clear cut as it once was. It is also a concentrated source of protein and other nutrients. However, there are other health issues specifically related to meat.

Meat contains multiple carcinogens, such as from environmental pollutants like PCBs, which are concentrated because it is further up the food chain[66]. As we saw, it also has various deleterious effects on the gut bacteria. Consumption of meat and other animal products cause an inflammatory response[25] which may be caused by endotoxins in the food, including bacteria that were killed in cooking but still cause an immune response[35].

Paleo advocates argue that despite containing significant amounts of meat, their diet is anti-inflammatory overall because it contains lots of anti-inflammatory plant foods, and minimizes dairy and grains, which are pro-inflammatory[19].

Fish

Fish are a good source of protein, and fatty fish like salmon
are a good source of omega3 fatty acids. The main health
concerns about fish are pollution including mercury and other
heavy metals. I recommend <u>Food, What The Heck Should I
Eat?</u>, by Dr. Mark Hyman, for good advice on healthy choices
for fish (as well as other animal foods)..

Legumes: Beans are Good- (if you are not allergic to them or have sensitivities to them)

One starchy food that is thought by most nutritionists to be
good is legumes, a source of low-glycemic carbs. They are
eaten in substantial amounts by all the world's healthiest
populations[178]. A study of the diets of elderly people of
various ethnic groups in four modern countries showed that
higher legume consumption is linked to increased longevity.
No other food considered, including meat, fruit, and
vegetables, correlated so strongly[22].

Beans are definitely a paleo food, there is abundant evidence
of their consumption in hunter gatherer societies as discussed
below ("Paleolithic Nutrition"). Some paleo advocates have
argued against legume consumption because they contain
phytic acid (also referred to as phytates), which can act as an
antinutrient, preventing the digestive system from absorbing
certain minerals.

One specific concern expressed is that this antinutrient effect may promote bone loss. But it turns out that higher phytate consumption correlates with better bone health, and it appears the mechanism may be that they block the formation of osteoclasts, the cells that break down bone cells, similar to anti-osteoporosis drugs like Fosamax but without side effects[230, 231]. Phytates are also an antioxidant, which has been shown to be beneficial in cancer prevention[52,53]. And phytic acid appears to only be harmful in excess, while some of us may be deficient in it. An article specifically on phytic acid stated "a subpopulation that might benefit from dietary phytic acid may be aging adults in the developed world[126]. Like me! For those still concerned about possible excess consumption of phytic acid, soaking legumes before cooking reduces its activity[130].

Beans also contain lectins, which are toxic, but are removed by soaking them overnight or cooking them long enough[155]. While lectins are toxic in high doses, there is evidence that low doses are beneficial, limiting tumor growth and helping with obesity[119].

Beans contain FODMAPs (short chain carbohydrates that are poorly absorbed in the small intestine)[188] which cause their flatulence infamy, although this too can be minimized by soaking. But some people are allergic to FODMAPs, kind of like the legume equivalent of gluten-sensitivity. It is best to avoid legumes if you are allergic, but they are healthy otherwise. This is why in chapter 4 it is recommended to carefully try reintroducing these kinds of foods after the reset. Even if you turn out not to be tolerant of beans, you may still tolerate a traditional product made from them like tofu or tempeh.

Soy

Specific concerns are raised about soy products because they are a source of phytoestrogens, which are mistakenly thought to have the same effect as the hormone estrogen. There are two types of estrogen receptor in the human body. Estrogen binds to the alpha receptor while phytoestrogens bind to the beta. These have the opposite effect on health: excess estrogen can cause breast cancer while phytoestrogens do not, in fact are protective against it[205]. And phytoestrogens do not have a feminizing effect on men ("man boobs")[103].

An additional health issue about soy is whether it is in a natural or highly processed form. Many commercial meat substitutes contain soy protein isolate, hydrolyzed soy protein, or textured soy protein. I was unable to find any research in the literature showing specific adverse health effects of these products, but they are extruded at high heat and the chemical hexane is used in the process so we are getting pretty far away from "minimally-processed".

I'm dubious about anything that's made in a processing facility that looks more like an oil refinery than a kitchen. If it's something that was traditionally processed, and you could make yourself if you wanted, I think it qualifies for minimally processed. Tofu and tempeh are traditional Asian foods made from soybeans. You can make tofu in your kitchen with soybeans and cheesecloth if you know what you're doing. Tempeh is made from fermented soybeans which is also apparently not hard to do yourself (http://store.organic-cultures.com/testpapts.html). I believe tofu and tempeh are healthy foods as long as you don't have any allergies to them. Products made from them are also healthy, although again I'd stick with organic sources like Tofurky.

Meat Substitutes

There are acceptable meat substitutes on the market (from the standpoint of minimally processed, no refined carbs) that are good vegan protein sources. I also recommend them for anyone trying to reduce meat consumption, although you can also cut back on meat by stretching it in recipes. Many meat substitutes are delicious and have a meat-like texture. Some of them are quite healthy, in my opinion, some not so much. The ones to avoid are made from soy protein isolates, discussed under soy. Anything made from tofu, tempeh, or seitan is minimally processed and is ok.

Because of the controversy over soy, and the fact that some people are allergic to soy, some commercial brands of meat substitutes are going with pea protein isolate, which, as near as I can tell, is a good alternative as long as it hasn't been chemically isolated. Unfortunately you can't always tell that from the label.

Seitan is a more modern term for a traditional Japanese product called Fu. It is made from vital wheat gluten, which is protein extracted from wheat. Seitan is pronounced like "satan" and from some of what you see about it on the internet, many feel that's appropriate. It certainly should be avoided by people with gluten sensitivity. But there is a gluten-free substitute called OrgraN from Australia, which you can get from Amazon. We discuss the pros and cons of grains below. For those without digestive issues with them, who think grains are ok in moderation, vital wheat gluten seems to be a healthy protein source.

Tofurky makes a substitute turkey from tofu, that's where they got their name. They have a meatless version of a Thanksgiving turkey feast that even includes little cutlets shaped like drumsticks. They also make ground beef and chicken substitutes. I mostly use their sausages which are delicious. They are made from organic tofu, expeller pressed canola oil, and spices. As we saw above, I consider expeller pressed canola a "yellow" food, its ok if it helps you to eat more "green" foods. Some of Tofurky's products also contain vital wheat gluten. I classify all of these as "yellow" foods, as long as you can tolerate gluten.

Sweet Earth makes "harmless ham", "benevolent bacon", and substitute meat strips, all from vital wheat gluten and other organic ingredients and "yellow" oils like evoo. Their veggie burgers are made with organic vegetable and grain ingredients and I consider a "green" food for those of us who can digest grains well.

A final caution about using meat substitutes: They don't always perform in recipes the way you think. My wife Karen makes a delicious spaghetti sauce with sausage and ground beef. I once tried substituting Tofurky sausage and their ground beef substitute. It was fine when I first made it. But when I tried to reheat the leftovers, the sausage and beef substitute had disappeared into the sauce, which now tasted like marinara sauce thickened with an unrecognizable paste. So if you try this, better to keep the meat substitute separate till the last minute.

Grains

Refined grains have the problem of causing a blood sugar spike as discussed in chapter 4. They are also inflammatory, and contribute to a number of health conditions such as obesity, diabetes, and heart disease. In contrast, minimally processed grains have a low glycemic load, and consumption of them is associated with lower risk of disease[39].

The same concerns are raised about antinutrients in grains, including phytic acid and lectins, which we already discussed under legumes. Grains are also suspected of contributing to leaky gut in susceptible people: "the consumption of wheat, but also other cereal grains, can contribute to the manifestation of chronic inflammation and autoimmune diseases by increasing intestinal permeability and initiating a pro-inflammatory immune response"[24], leading to conditions including Crohn's disease and other inflammatory bowel diseases, and irritable bowel syndrome.

In addition, some people are allergic or have sensitivities to grains, like gluten sensitivity, or in its more severe form celiac diseases. There is evidence that gluten sensitivity is worse for modern hybridized wheat, so alternative grains or "ancient grains" may cause less of a problem[153]. There is also some evidence that yeast is also a trigger for inflammation in Crohn's disease, so some people may be able to tolerate foods with grains as long as they don't contain yeast[213].

It also needs to be pointed out that animal products are also an important factor in promoting Crohn's disease, and for many people a plant-based diet is more beneficial than avoiding grains[214]. Minimally-processed grains are a healthy food as long as you are not one of the people with these digestive issues. If you suspect you have sensitivities to grains, you can try eliminating and reintroducing them, and get tested for gluten sensitivity.

There are a lot of gluten free and "pseudo-grain" options available if they are a problem for you. One of the major benefits claimed for whole grains is fiber, but there are many grain-free high-fiber sources, including: broccoli, raspberries, blackberries, avocados, flaxseeds, chia seeds, pears, apples, strawberries, figs, almonds, and buckwheat (a pseudo-grain made from a seed). Buckwheat is a staple in Eastern Europe, where it is called kasha, and in Japan, it is used to make soba noodles.

Sustainable Agriculture

In addition to the health reasons for following a wfpb diet, many choose to reduce animal food consumption for reasons such as wanting to avoid inhumane treatment of animals, or because of religious belief. I respect these reasons, but they can cause the discussion about animal products to be more heated than other issues. Brian Kateman, in his book <u>The Reduceitarian Solution</u>[74], suggests that rather than present it as a black and white issue of vegans vs meat eaters, it would help if it were just stated that everyone could consider cutting back on animal products, which sounds reasonable to me.

There are also environmental issues. Animal agriculture, especially modern factory farming, is inefficient compared to growing plants. Traditionally, animals were grazed on land that was less suitable for farming like hillsides, but modern large scale animal production uses large amounts of prime land. Many are concerned that this type of practice is not sustainable for feeding the earth's large and growing population. It's not just animal agriculture that's inefficient. Giant fields of commodity crops like corn, wheat, potatoes, and soybeans are planted just to make snack foods, for example. So it helps to avoid processed foods, buy sustainably raised plant and animal foods, as well as consider "reduceitarianism".

Current (or recent) Healthy Populations

There are multiple populations around the world following a traditional lifestyle and diet that have much lower incidence of "diseases of civilization", and better health and longevity, than the average for modern western countries. In addition to the diet, they all have good social support and care and respect for elders, and are very physically active.

The areas where they live have been referred to as "blue zones"[178]. These populations eat a diet that is largely whole food plant based (wfpb), consuming relatively few calories from animal products (the percentage of calories from animal foods ranges from 0 to about 15%). They do not eat modern processed foods, but instead eat lots of fruit, vegetables, nuts, and legumes. All eat some grains, some minimally processed, others, like the Okinawans, eat white rice, but not as a high percentage of their diet. All of these populations tend to have total cholesterol < 150, ldl < 70, and low triglycerides.

Most of them are rural, with the exception of the Seventh Day Adventists in Loma Linda, California, who are in an urban area. All the blue zone populations have access to modern medicine, so infant mortality and infectious disease rates are low.

There also may be other healthy populations that are eating a higher meat and low carb diet. I discuss the examples of the Inuits and the Masai below. The evidence for them is a little murkier. The Masai, especially, appear to be in good health but do not have good longevity. It could be higher if corrected for infant mortality rate and infectious disease, but I have not seen data for that. This does not mean it is not possible to be healthy and long-lived on these diets, but we don't have the evidence to prove it.

Proof that the health benefits of the blue-zone populations are not genetic comes from members of these populations that abandon the old ways or move away and adapt more western lifestyles. Sadly this is increasingly true in Okinawa where the younger people are adopting a western diet and lifestyle, and their health and longevity is plummeting[132]. Another example is rural Chinese who are healthy and long-lived on a wfpb diet, then migrate to the city. They adopt a modern diet and lifestyle and become much less healthy.

Several changes occur when the traditional ways are abandoned, including:

- Consumption of junk (modern processed food) goes way up
- Consumption of animal products increases
- Physically activity decreases
- Social support probably decreases
- Stress levels are probably higher

The story of these populations and others like them is one of the main motivations for the wfpb diet. But it should be noted it does not prove, by itself, that is the animal consumption that is the culprit in the Western diet, because there are multiple differences between the traditional and modern diets and lifestyles. Another point is that with the exception of Seventh Day Adventist vegans, who avoid animal products for religious reasons, these groups traditionally all eat some animal products, though much less than in the SAD. One reason more meat is not eaten is that, like everyone except the wealthy until modern times, animal products are a luxury. When meat is eaten, it is used more like a condiment except on feast occasions.

A Closer Look at The Blue Zones

Dan Buettner's book <u>The Blue Zones</u> describes healthy and long-lived populations living in local regions around the world he calls the "Blue Zones". All of these populations get a lot of physical activity, have strong family ties, a high level of social engagement, and have low rates of smoking.

- Okinawa (Japan). The staple of the diet is local sweet potatoes, with garden vegetables, a local bitter melon called goya that has high antioxidant content, tofu, miso soup, white rice, fish, and occasional pork. Fish and meat total about 15% of the diet. Okinawans following the traditional lifestyle remain lean for life and have very good longevity. It is a part of traditional Okinawan culture to not overeat, instead stopping when pleasantly satisfied. Between this and the quality diet, the Okinawan lifestyle leads to healthy aging[161].
- Sardinia (Italy). The Blue Zone here is a subset of the population that lives in an isolated cluster of villages. The locals eat whole grain bread, beans, garden vegetables, and milk and cheese from their goats (they are shepherds on steep hillsides), with meat as an "accent food". The goats graze on a local plant that is thought to give the milk more health properties. They drink a local wine that is extra-rich in flavonoids, which have anti-inflammatory properties.
- Nicoya (Costa Rica). The local water has a naturally high calcium content. Food includes maize, rice, beans, locally grown fruits (some exotic and antioxidant rich), vegetables (including local wild plants), some milk curd, eggs, and meat once or twice a week.

- Ikaria (Greece): Their diet has been precisely documented by Greek researchers, with these statistics: 3700 calories per day, about 72% carb, 11% protein, 17% fat, and 13% calories from animal products. The food is vegetables (including an astonishing 150 local wild greens), fruits, legumes, potatoes, meat and fish, olive oil, pasta and rice. Grains are about 4% of the calories, legumes about 7%. Probably at least half their protein is from meat and fish. Note how high the calorie count is. The estimated calorie need for a moderately active American adult is 2600 for males and 2000 for females[174]. Something tells me, since they are lean, that the Ikarians must move a lot more than us!

The Seventh-day Adventists in Loma Linda, California. They have been studied the most thoroughly and their diet is described next.

The Adventist Health Study

One of the most interesting studies of the health aspects of the vegan/vegetarian diets is the Adventist health study[114]. Many of the healthy wfpb populations described above are rural, consuming traditional diets. You might think "I could be healthy too if I lived on the gorgeous Greek island of Ikaria". But the Seventh Day Adventists studied were from Loma Linda California, near Riverside, which, complete with freeways, is definitely not rural. There were several studies of this population, leading to dozens of papers in peer-reviewed journals. Members of this religion have principles that affect their diet strongly, including:

- An interpretation of a bible verse (Genesis 1:29) to mean we should abstain from eating meat. Some take it as an injunction against all animal products.
- Taking the biblical teaching that our bodies are temples seriously, which leads to various good health habits like good diet, not smoking, and staying physically active.

Researchers separated Adventists into 3 groups, all of whom practice nonsmoking and good physical activity habits, and follow a diet healthier than the SAD. The first group is vegan, the second lacto-vegetarian (vegan plus dairy products), and the third also eat some meat. They are all healthier than the general American population, but the vegans are the healthiest, in fact they are some of the healthiest and longest-living people on the planet. The lacto-vegetarians are somewhat less healthy than the vegans, and those who consume meat are the least healthy of the three.

This might lead someone to conclude "Plant based is best, adding dairy is a little worse, eating meat is worst of all". But that is debatable. Since the interpretation of the first Adventist guideline is a little ambiguous, we can argue that the vegans and lacto-vegetarians both feel they are following that to the letter. The meat eating group is clearly violating that guideline, though. Maybe they are a bit looser in general, and not following the second guideline as well either (perhaps they eat a little more refined food and don't exercise as much).

There is not enough information in the study to tell. There are also some clues from other populations like the Okinawans and Ikarians, who eat some meat but little or no dairy, and are also healthy with good longevity. There is also a pesco-vegetarian subset of Adventists (vegan except for some fish consumption) that has slightly higher longevity than the vegan group[114].

The remarkable health and longevity of the vegans is still an important takeaway from the Adventist study. Because of the second guideline above, it is likely they follow a wfpb/vegan diet, minimizing consumption of refined foods. I can confirm this anecdotally, because in the vegetarian days of my youth, I used a great cookbook by the Seventh-day Adventist author Rosalie Hurd called the Ten Talents Cookbook, which is still in print[200]. She definitely emphasized whole foods and healthy eating all throughout that book. Mrs. Hurd won the Mrs. America cooking contest (which is judged on flavor), competing against non-vegetarian cooks. The winning recipe was in her book. It didn't turn out very well when I made it: I am most assuredly not an award winning cook.

Rural Africans

Many rural Africans practice a combination of subsistence farming and gathering. Because these are not affluent populations, consumption of animal products is relatively low, and a variety of plant foods are consumed. There is much lower incidence of modern degenerative diseases like heart diseases, hypertension, diabetes, and cancer compared to urban societies not eating a traditional diet[158].

In 1929, researchers measured the blood pressure of a thousand people in rural Kenya eating a diet mostly of maize, legumes, vegetables, fruits, and wild greens. It was low by modern standards (typically around 110/70) and did not increase with age[199]. It's interesting that the increase of blood pressure with age is still referred to by the obsolete medical term "essential hypertension": It was thought until not that long ago that blood pressure had to increase with age because the arteries "inevitably" get stiffer so more pressure is needed to get the same blood flow. For a long time it was thought that the "normal" value for systolic (the upper number) blood pressure was 100 plus age. So my "normal" would be 165! Clearly increase in blood pressure was not "essential" for rural Kenyans, and that has been known since 1929.

In various parts of rural Africa on a similar diet, there is also very low incidence of heart disease, obesity, and diabetes, and cancer[158].

The Masai

The Masai belong to a special population that does not follow the typical rural African diet. They are a legendary East African people whose men traditionally protected their cattle herds from lions with spears. You can't get much braver than that. It is commonly believed the men also traditionally consumed large amounts of meat, milk, and blood. In 1964, 400 of the men were studied and found to have low cholesterol, no incidence of high blood pressure, and no abnormalities in ekg tests[91]. This implies a low level of heart disease, although the ekg testing is not conclusive, as it is possible to have coronary artery disease without ekg abnormalities.

In 1972, it was confirmed that for the Masai men "intake of animal fat exceeds that of American men". Fifty deceased Masai men were autopsied, and it was found that there was extensive atherosclerosis but "very few complicated lesions", and "the coronary arteries showed intimal thickening by atherosclerosis which equaled that of old U.S. men. The Masai vessels enlarge with age to more than compensate for this disease. It is speculated that the Masai are protected from their atherosclerosis by physical fitness which causes their coronary vessels to be capacious"[92].

Not as much was known about atherosclerosis vs. atherothrombosis in 1972. It is possible that if the autopsies were repeated today, the "few complicated lesions" might mean that the atherosclerosis observed was stable plaque, and not likely to lead to atherothrombosis (bursting of the "pimple", as discussed above). So the speculation that "the Masai are protected from their atherosclerosis by physical fitness which causes their coronary vessels to be capacious" might still be valid. But it does not mean they were protected from heart attacks (they didn't need such protection because atherothrombosis was unlikely), but possibly their enlarged arteries due to their fitness protected them from other conditions like angina.

The Masai have poor longevity compared to typical modern cultures. Hopefully they will get better access to modern medicine which could help with infectious disease and infant mortality, improving their longevity. But we don't yet have proof.

Alaskan Inuits/Greenland Eskimos

It is commonly believed that Inuits have low incidence of heart disease despite a traditional diet high in animal products and high in saturated fat (a common theory is that their high Omega-3 consumption due to eating lots of fish is protective). This appears, however, to have no scientific foundation. Researchers Bang and Dyerberg visited Greenland Eskimos multiple times in the 1960s, and reported they had low incidence of cardiovascular disease, which is the basis for the belief.

But from a recent literature review: "The fact is that Bang and Dyerberg did not examine the cardiovascular status of the Greenland Eskimos" and "Instead, they relied mainly on Annual Reports produced by the Chief Medical Officer (CMO) in Greenland for the years 1963-1967 and 1973-1976" which were shown to have limited validity for verifying cardiovascular status. Further "the prevalence of heart disease among Eskimos in Greenland and other Inuit populations in Canada and the US is similar or higher compared to that of non-Eskimo/Caucasian populations"[45].

The Greenland Eskimos and Alaskan Inuits are in fact rare populations for which switching to a modern diet lowered their risk of dying from heart disease: "The decrease in mortality from IHD in Greenland since 1965 is surprising in view of the rapid westernization of the country during the same period. A similar trend was present among Alaska Natives"[5]. And autopsies of mummified Alaskan Inuit bodies from over 500 years ago showed significant atherosclerosis[167].

Paleolithic Nutrition

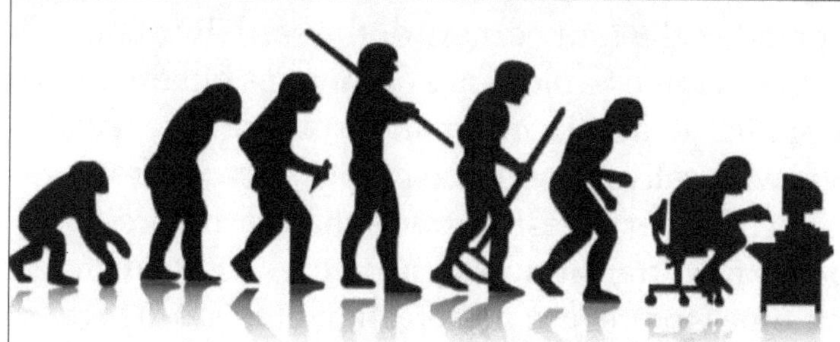

I have seen exaggerated dietary claims based on evolutionary reasoning from different viewpoints, vegans claiming it shows we were herbivores, paleo advocates that we evolved eating a lot of meat, and low-carb advocates that we evolved for a million years eating low carb. The truth is a bit murkier, as we'll see. Exactly what we evolved on is controversial. But it is clear from the fossil record that pre-agriculture hunter gatherers were robust and in good health, and I think a lot can be inferred about healthy eating from their various diets, which ranged from high plant content/low animal to low plant/high animal, depending on the environment they were in.

For about 99% of our evolution humans were primates, eating a diet with a very high percentage of plant foods[105]. The first Humans (Homo Sapiens) appeared about 200,000 years ago in Africa, and spread to the four corners of the earth by about 40,000 years ago[31]. Homo Sapiens are omnivores but are more anatomically similar to herbivores than carnivores: we have alkaline saliva, with salivary amylase to digest starch from plant foods, much longer digestive tracts than carnivores[68], and much longer food transit times (carnivores have much shorter transit times to prevent putrefaction of meat). There have been counter-arguments about the human digestive tract vs carnivores[1], but flaws have been pointed out in the measurements used, and upon closer examination the human digestive tract appears to most closely resemble that of frugivores (fruit eaters)[68], which makes sense since other primates eat diets high in fruit.

We do have some distinctions from herbivores, for example we are poor at synthesizing the amino acid taurine, which is a carnivore trait because taurine is readily available from animal sources[19]. Other examples include different populations having different numbers of copies of a gene that involved in digesting starch: "individuals from populations with high-starch diets have on average more AMY1 copies than those with traditionally low-starch diets"[120]. Rather than showing we *evolved* to eat meat, these appear to be more like "tweaks" to a basic herbivore anatomy that *allow* us to eat meat. That doesn't prove that eating meat is not good for us, but it weakens any argument that we evolved to eat meat.

An important controversy is over what type of food "made us human". This dispute is over what enabled the large expansion in brain size that occurred in our hominid ancestors over a few hundred thousand years, leading to Homo Sapiens. It is well accepted that since a larger brain requires a lot more energy, our ancestors probably found a novel source of calories.

The two main candidates are meat[1] and cooked starches[60], especially tubers[94]. Humans have much smaller jaw muscles than other primates, and are missing the sagittal crest on our skulls to anchor larger jaw muscles. It seems reasonable to assume this is because humans no longer had to chew for hours on raw starchy foods, as other primates do. Instead, cooking "predigested" starch for us[165]. That is a controversial point, and I'm not sure what percentage of evolutionary biologists believe that the novel food source that accounts for the evolutionary brain growth was meat or cooked starch, or a combination.

But I don't think the paleo diet needs to be based on how we evolved. Instead, in my opinion, the most compelling argument is to examine the apparent health as well as the diet of hunter gatherer populations before the invention of agriculture. When Homo Sapiens left Africa and spread all over the planet, it was during the last ice age, so places like Europe and North America were cold and had large mammals, and the inhabitants adapted to hunting. The fossil record for robust hunter gatherers is largely from this period[31].

As for the composition of the pre-agricultural diet, examination of coprolite, or fossilized feces (sounds like a fun job) shows hunter gatherers had a high fiber diet, so they consumed a lot of plant foods. They could also have eaten a lot of animal foods as well, that is not conclusive from the fossil record. Many wild plant foods are highly fibrous but not calorically dense, so a high plant food volume could have been eaten without necessarily contributing a high percentage of the calories in the diet.

Fossil evidence shows that these people were lean, fit, and robust, with no "diseases of civilization". In contrast, evidence from agriculture civilizations often show shorter stature and poorer teeth, and evidence of deficiency diseases[31]. The agricultural people may well have been protein deficient and had very little variety in their diet compared to hunter gatherers. Clearly, switching from a diet with a variety of nutritious plant and animal foods to one that relied on a few staple foods like grains, with inadequate protein, as was done in cultures practicing intensive agriculture, was not a good move. So it is reasonable to argue that relying on foods like grains as the staple of the diet is not optimal for health. But we do not have evidence from the fossil record, nor from contemporary hunter-gatherers, of longevity past 60 on a hunter-gatherer diet. That does not mean it is not possible, with access to modern medicine to address infectious disease and infant mortality, but there are no data to prove it.

There is a fascinating history of hunter gatherers in North America in <u>The Art and Science of Low-Carbohydrate Living</u> including the "bison people". Eating a diet high in meat, low in carbs, and without enough fat, if not done properly, can lead to a deadly condition called protein toxicity (also known as "rabbit starvation" or "Mal de Caribou"). This can happen in cold climates, especially in the winter when not enough plant foods are available, if the animal sources of food are too lean. The bison people made ingenious adaptations to obtain enough fat. There is also a description of a valuable trade good, candlefish oil, which was harvested along the Pacific coast for at least 10000 years, and had a fatty acid profile as healthy as olive oil. We also know that Native Americans relied on pemmican[176], a high fat food made from meat and fat. This was also an important trade item. From these examples and similar ones from Europe, it is clear that ancestors from this period in colder regions were getting a lot of calories from animal foods.

What is not certain is whether the diet high in animal foods was what they evolved on, or was an adaptation to the environments they found themselves in after they left Africa. In the same era, those in more temperate or tropical locales adapted to eating less animal foods and more plant foods.

Estimates of the Paleo Diet From Contemporary Hunters and Gatherers

Further evidence about hunter-gatherer diets comes from examining the diets of hunters and gatherers still following their traditional lifestyle in the modern world, which were more prevalent as late as the 1970s[30].

Drs. Boyd Eaton and Melvin Konner published a paper on Paleolithic nutrition in 1985 which estimated the average hunter-gatherer population consumed about 35% of their calories from animal foods, 65% plant. This was based on data in the Ethnographic Atlas, a database on 1167 societies, published by George P. Murdock in multiple installments in the journal Ethnology from 1962 to 1980[109]. In addition to the average, they estimated a variation of percentage of calories in the diet of different societies from 90% plant/10% animal to 10% plant/90% animal depending on the environment[30].

Dr. Loren Cordain made a detailed statistical analysis of the data in the Ethnographic Atlas and came up with a different estimate, that most hunter gatherers societies would have gotten more than 50% of their calories from animal foods, and would have consumed a relatively high amount of protein and lower amount of carbohydrates[18].

Using the data in the Ethnographic Atlas for the purpose of estimating diet is controversial: it was "written by ethnographers or others with disparate backgrounds, rarely interested in diet per se or trained in dietary collection techniques."[105]. Also the results in the atlas could have been skewed "because most of the ethnographers were male, they often did not associate with women, who typically collect and process plant resources", and most hunter-gathering societies remaining by the 20th century "had been displaced to marginal environments."

The evidence in support of any single version of the paleo diet is controversial. I think it is more widely agreed that there were a variety of pre-agricultural diets, ranging from higher meat in colder regions to higher plant sources in more temperate zones. It is likely most of these diets included:

1. A variety of plant foods.
2. Minimal consumption of grains: grains such as wild
   rice in North America and wild barley and oats in
   prehistoric Greece[56] were available, but would have
   been harder to gather, so probably would have made
   up a smaller percentage of the diet.
3. Little or no dairy.
4. Animal foods including meat, eggs, fish, and insects.
   Meat from wild game would have been much leaner
   than modern domesticated animals and had a better fat
   profile (see discussion of Omega3 above). Paleo authors
   recommend grass-fed beef and pasture raised chickens
   to address this, but the fat content is still higher than
   wild game. However, the counterarguments are that
   organ meats would have been a prized source of fat,
   and the ingenuity describe above to obtain sufficient
   fat[121].

Some paleo authors claim that legumes were not consumed in
hunter-gatherer times but there is plenty of evidence to
contradict that, including lentil and pea consumption in
prehistoric Greece[56], substantial consumption of tsin beans by
the !Kung in Africa[80], and acacia seeds (which are a legume)
by Australian aborigines[86], and fossil evidence of legume (and
grain) consumption on Neanderthal teeth[64].

It seems you can be eating a variety of amounts of plant and
animal foods and still be "eating paleo". This is also discussed
in detail in Rob Wolfs' book <u>Wired to Eat</u>.

Small Scale Agriculture

The advent of agriculture in many regions of the world
spawned large civilizations based on large scale farming.
These often relied on few, or even one, staple of the diet
("daily bread", corn, potatoes, etc.) and had little variety, and
were probably deficient in protein. And this led to poor health
compared to hunter gatherers.

But some populations continued their hunter-gatherer
lifestyle, supplemented by small scale agriculture, so they still
got plenty of protein and a good variety of food sources.
Examples include Native Americans growing some maize or
planting orchards, or other cultures planting tubers. The
evidence is that these cultures were just as healthy as hunter
gatherers[177]. And most of the rural "blue zone" populations in
the world today, that experience the best health and longevity
known, also practice small scale agriculture[178]. This may be
considered "eating early neo" instead of "eating paleo" but it
is still healthy.

Is it All a Paleofantasy?

The paleo diet has been criticized by some evolutionary
biologists recently. Dismissing it as a "paleofantasy" seems a
bit harsh, but they make some valid points, especially about
the assumption that there is only one version and it has *no*
grains, and *no* legumes.

Paleofantasy is the title of Dr. Marlene Zuk's book. If you read
the book carefully she does not dismiss the whole concept of
getting clues about what might be healthy by examining what
hunter gatherers ate. But she has three main objections:

- Some proponents of the paleo diet present a single version of the diet as the universal ideal diet. She points out that there were many varieties of hunter gatherer diets.
- She objects to viewing the advent of agriculture as a disaster and what she sees as the fantasy of abandoning civilization and returning to the hunter gatherer lifestyle. She argues there was no point in the past at which we were perfectly adapted to the environment. But despite this objection she does agree that "the past can inform the present" so we can get clues for healthy eating from what worked well in the past vs what is not working well now, like modern processed food.
- A main basis of the paleo diet is the "discordance hypothesis", originally proposed by Dr. Boyd Eaton[30], that all the lifestyle changes that have occurred since the advent of agriculture and civilization were very rapid on an evolutionary time scale, and that we have not had time to evolve to them. We evolved to be the guy with the spear in the cartoon above, but in the blink of an eye we're hunched over the computer or worse yet, sitting in a lazy-boy recliner eating junk food. But actually organisms can adapt quickly when their environment changes, which is Dr. Zuk's specialty. She gives some fascinating examples of rapid adaptation to environmental changes in insects and animals. As for humans, there are multiple cases like a genetic variation that allows some of us to digest lactose as adults, and the adaptation to resist malaria, that have occurred after the advent of agriculture.

But I don't think the fact that we have done some evolving since 10,000 years ago invalidates the paleo idea. She points out elsewhere in the book that evolutionary changes are often not perfect designs, but compromises. Our spines show evidence that they evolved at a time when we were still knuckle draggers (actually they also have features dating back to fish). They are not ideally suited for us to be upright which can lead to back issues, but becoming upright was an evolutionary advantage.

Another good example of a compromise is the adaptation to malaria in Africa, the sickle cell mutation. If you get one copy of the sickle cell gene it makes you more resistant to malaria, but if you get two copies, it causes sickle cell anemia, a terrible disease. This is clearly not a perfect solution but a compromise. But to me these examples still make the discordance hypothesis valid. Yes it is possible for us to evolve so we would be better able to digest twinkies, but that adaptation would likely be a compromise with side effects. Isn't it better to just eat healthy foods and avoid the need for that adaptation?

Dr. Zuk also makes a distinction between horticulture and intensive agriculture: We didn't go straight from being hunter-gatherers to living in cities eating mostly bread. There were hunter-gatherers who remained healthy and fit, who supplemented their diet by planting some tubers or other small crops with sticks. I discussed this above under "small scale agriculture".

The Paleo diet was also discussed in a Ted talk by Dr. Christine Wariner, (www.youtube.com/watch?v=BMOjVYgYaG8&t=21s). She too objected to the paleo diet in the form of high meat, no grain, no legumes, no dairy, and argued that the fossil record does not support this: hunter gatherers instead ate a variety of foods depending on their region. She also made an interesting argument that the modern versions of foods that are allowed on the paleo diet, like veggies and fruits, bear no relation to their wild Paleolithic cousins. Some of the salad greens we eat, for example, are bitter and almost indigestible in their wild state. Wild almonds are poisonous (contain too much cyanide). She wonders why we are allowed to eat modern versions of foods like these, highly modified by centuries of farming practices, and call that paleo.

She concludes with some lessons we can learn from what the fossil record does show: There is no one correct diet, but we should eat a diverse amount of whole foods (such as a variety of fruits and veggies), and avoid processed foods. This is not incompatible with a more flexible definition of paleo.

Proponents of the paleo diet convincingly argue that the advent of agriculture caused a major change in our diets that was incompatible with what we evolved to thrive on. But an even bigger change occurred more recently, with the advent of modern processed foods. And that has clearly not worked out well either.

Diet, Fat Adaptation, And Athletic Performance

Some authors claim that our bodies have a "preferred fuel" which may be fat or carbs depending on who you listen to. But our bodies are really "flex fuel" vehicles. They have a small fuel tank containing "higher octane" fuel (glycogen), and a much larger tank containing a slightly "lower octane" fuel (fat). I'll explain why fat can be called "lower octane" below.

The body wants to use the abundantly available fuel, fat, at lower intensities so it can go farther. At higher intensities which tend to be shorter activities, it wants to burn more carbs because it lets you go harder with the same amount of oxygen. By "carbs", I'm really referring to glycogen in the muscles and liver, which is how the body stores carbs.

The figures shown below are for hypothetical athletes with varying levels of fat adaptation. Some examples from actual athletes are given in Dr. Grant Schofield's book <u>What The Fat? Sports Performance: Leaner, Fitter, Faster on Low-Carb Healthy Fat</u>.

The first figure shows how carb and fat burning varies with exercise intensity, for a person with a well-functioning metabolism. At low intensities, mostly fat is burned and very little carbs. At high intensity, the body has to work hard to supply enough oxygen to working muscles, so more carbs are burned and less fat:

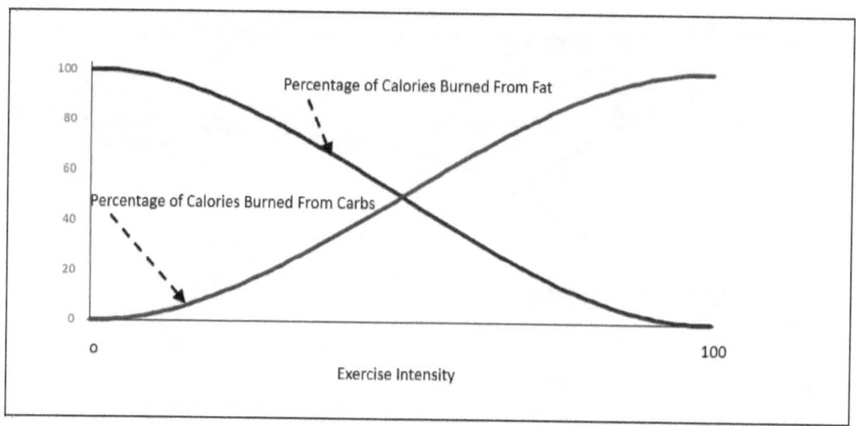

Next we see a person that is poorly fat adapted. Even at rest and for low intensity activities, a significant amount of carbs are being burned:

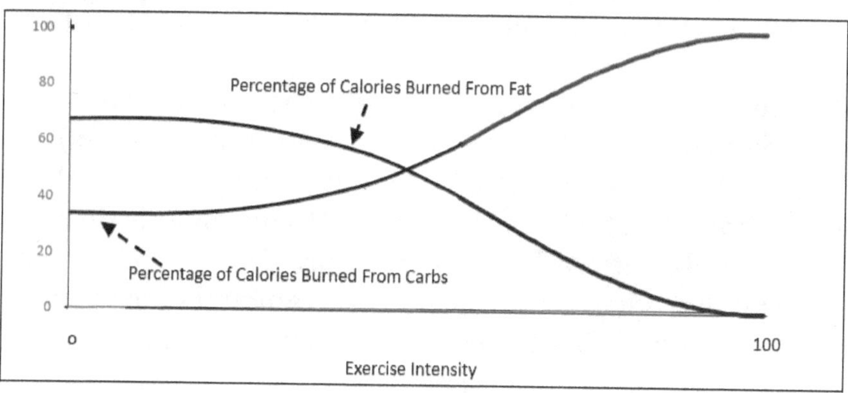

This is probably typical for a person with a dysfunctional metabolism. The reset should go a long way to fix this. It also helps to get aerobically fitter by doing more training. A specific training trick that helps is not taking in calories while working out at low to moderate intensities, especially in longer sessions. We'll revisit that in more detail below.

Next we see a person that is highly fat adapted, and on a low-carb diet, so this person burns more fat even at higher intensities:

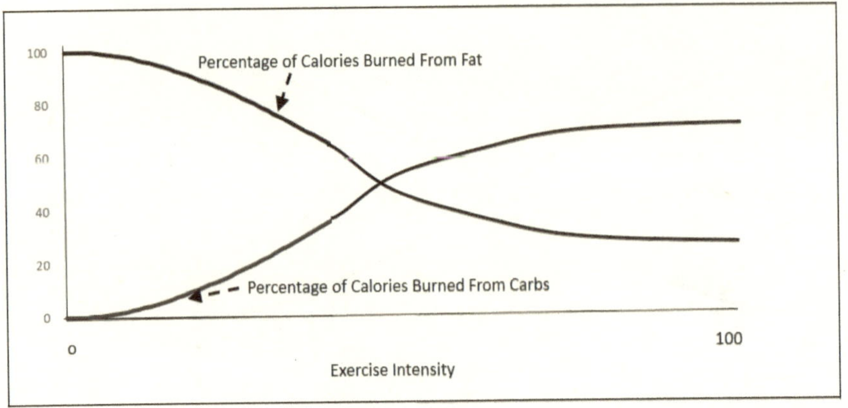

At first glance this seems to be advantageous, as is claimed by low-carb authors. Our bodies can only store about 2000 calories of glycogen, but even the leanest people store more than 10 times that amount as fat. That means you can exercise a lot longer if you are a "fat burner", even at higher intensities.

But there's a tradeoff. On a low carb diet the body actually down-regulates the ability to burn carbs, so at high intensities, it is as much "poorly carb adapted" as it is "fat adapted". This means there is less fuel available for fast twitch muscle fibers, which can only burn carbs. Also, it requires 7½% more oxygen to burn fat than glycogen[201], so at a given amount of oxygen intake, performance is a bit less burning fat, which is where I got the "lower octane" from. This is basic physiology, but is often not mentioned by low-carb authors.

The question is whether it is a good trade-off to burn more fat a higher intensities like in the chart above. If you try to do a longer event at higher intensity, like the marathon and beyond, it might be good to burn more fat and less glycogen, even if it's lower octane fuel, to keep from running out of glycogen.

For many people, enough glycogen is being burned at marathon pace to empty out the small tank by around mile 20. So we "hit the wall" (also known as "bonking") at this point, slowing down considerably (a lot more than 7½%) and feeling awful. The feeling is because neither the brain nor the muscles are getting enough sugar. Even short of bonking, having low glycogen stores can make us feel grumpy, or "hangry", as some people describe it (for the combination of hungry and angry).

One way to stave this off is to "carbo-load", or eat a higher carb diet leading up to the event so your body's glycogen tanks are full to the brim. The problem with that is that your body stores water along with glycogen, so this makes you weigh more at the race and you can feel a bit bloated. And extra weight is payload, slowing you down. A second way to fight the dreaded "wall" is taking in calories during the event by using energy drinks like Gatorade or energy gels, and it can be a trade-off between bringing in enough fuel and not causing gastric distress.

Being adapted to using more of a lower octane fuel at marathon pace, so that you don't run out of glycogen, avoids the need to carbo-load and risk gastric distress by taking in calories on the run. That sounds like not such a bad bargain, which is why participants in longer events are becoming interested in low-carb eating.

Bonking is even more of an issue for ultra-marathon running or longer events like ironman triathlons because it's difficult to take in enough calories during the event. On recreational outings like century rides or long hikes, lasting several hours, it's relatively easy to take in enough food. If you've watched long bike races like the Tour de France you've probably seen the "feed zone" where the cyclists are handed bags full of food to keep them going.

The first glimmer I heard that a nutritional approach to fat adaptation might work for longer events was the performance of Mark Allen, 6 time winner of the Hawaii Ironman. He was following the nutritional strategy of Dr. Phil Maffetone, which at the time included a diet of 40% carbs, 30% fat, 30% protein[99]. By eating only 40% carbs, there is no way he could take in enough carbs to finish an 8 hour event without bonking, according to conventional nutritional wisdom. The logical answer is he didn't have to, because even at the elite pace needed to win an Ironman, Allen was getting a higher percentage of energy from fat than sugar- he was more fat-adapted than his competitors.

More recently, fat adaptation has become a hot topic, but the emphasis is often on keto-adaptation[121], which is having your body adapt to being in a state of nutritional ketosis, explained in chapter 4. Some significant results have been obtained: most notably keto-adapted runner Timothy Olson won the Western States 100 mile ultramarathon twice, and set the course record in 2013 of just under 15 hours. That is impressive, but Scott Jurek won Western States a record 7 straight times and was a previous record holder, and from his book Eat to Live, it is clear his diet was whole food plant based and not low carb. Olson's record was broken by Jim Walmsley in 2018, who was also not a low-carb eater[209].

The disadvantage of eating a low-carb diet is that high end performance is not as good, as mentioned above, making it seem a better strategy for ultraendurance events than for shorter events. But recently the strategy of "train low, race high" has been developed- use the ketogenic diet while training but take in extra carbs for your event, boosting high end performance[54], which seems to work well for some people. I haven't heard how short of an event you can be competitive in using this approach.

One thing I haven't seen explained satisfactorily is what the advantage is of going all the way to a ketogenic diet. We started with having to drink a lot of Gatorade and eat little gel packets just to get through a marathon, then flipped all the way over to an extremely low-carb diet. Isn't there a happy medium in between? We know that Mark Allen was fat-adapted but not on a ketogenic diet so the answer appears to be yes. What benefit does the ketogenic approach have over this more moderate approach? Dr. Grant Schofield is an MD in New Zealand, and also a triathlete, who advocates a restricted carb but not ketogenic diet[136]. He claims that while the ketogenic diet does lead to fat adaptation, you can also get fat adapted, but more slowly, without going into ketosis. And there can be some unpleasant side effects of transitioning into ketosis that are avoided with a more moderate approach.

We already discussed the "lower octane" effect of fat, that it takes 7½% more oxygen to get the same amount of energy from fat as from carbs, so while cruising at the same percentage of max oxygen uptake, the more fat-adapted athlete is slower. That is the downside to low carb eating and fat adaptation for athletic performance, as explained on nutritionist Jeff Rothschild's website[168] and in exercise physiologist Dr. Owen Anderson's <u>Running Science</u>. This is not just a theoretical result, there is evidence of degraded race performance in athletes who improve their fat adaptation by eating low carb[12]. The "train low, race high" strategy doesn't fix this because low-carb diets have a negative effect on the ability to use carbs after fat adaptation[148].

But there are some techniques to becoming somewhat more fat adapted without eating a low carb diet. Eating a diet of alkaline producing foods like fruits and veggies (scientific term is "low Potential renal acid load" or low PRAL) enhances fat adaptation[13]. Meat, dairy, and grains are pro-acidic, so cutting back on one or more of these helps. In vegan or wfpb, meat and dairy are eliminated or drastically reduced, while in paleo, dairy and grains are, so either of diets these can be alkaline.

You can also avoid taking in calories during long training sessions. In a comment to his post about low carb and fat adaptation, I asked Jeff Rothschild whether doing this type of technique while eating higher carb the rest of the time would have the same negative performance effects mentioned above, and he replied "Doing a few sessions per week with little or no fuel in the tank won't have negative effects on carb utilization". He and Conrad Earnest discuss various dietary manipulations and how they affect fat adaptation and athletic performance in detail in ref. 217.

I eat a diet with very few refined carbs but plenty of carbs from whole foods as discussed in "my eating story". I don't usually measure, but I estimate I eat about 50% carbs, higher than the 40% of Mark Allen but less than the 60% often recommended in nutrition suggestions for endurance athletes. I can go at least 4 hours at a brisk cruising pace without "bonking". When on a group bike ride or hike, whenever there's a break, I see others reaching for power-bars, trail mix, etc., which I don't find necessary. And at the end I am not "hangry" or desperate to "carb reload". So I must be pretty well fat adapted. Aside from eating an alkaline diet, the main trick I've used is that I don't take in any carbs during my workouts, including my longest workouts of the week, so my body gets used to not getting its sugar tank topped off.

Four hours is about the longest activity I do these days so this is enough for me. I would guess that before doing these adaptations I probably could only cruise for a little over 2 hours without bonking unless I took in carbs along the way.

Suggested Reading

Inspiration

- <u>The Anna Meares Story -When Courage Triumphs Over Disaster</u>, Anna Meares. Inspiring description of Anna's comeback after she broke her neck in a track cycling crash. After a tough rehab she courageously "got back on the horse" and started racing again, going on to win gold in London, 2012.
- <u>Iron Heart: The True Story of How I Came Back from the Dead</u>, Brian Boyle. Brian was so badly injured when hit by a car on his bike that during emergency surgery some major organs, including his heart, had to be put back in the right position. He lost 100 pounds during his recovery. After an amazing rehab he went on to complete an ironman triathlon.
- <u>Old Lady on the Trail: Triple Crown at 76</u>, Mary Davison. Mary is the oldest woman, and as far as I know the oldest person, to have completed hiking all 3 of the US's premier trails- Appalachian, Continental Divide, and Pacific Crest. This is despite overcoming some age- related issues.

- <u>Running The Red Line</u>, Julie Carter. Julie is a medical doctor who is also a passionate fell runner. I find fell running fascinating. In my running days I used to love going fast down trails, but fell runners go fast in places where there are no trails. Julie overcame a major congenital back problem to become age-group British fell running champion in her 50s, and also completed major ultraendurance challenges like the 24 hour Bob Graham round.

- <u>Operation Ironman: One Man's Four Month Journey from Hospital Bed to Ironman Triathlon</u>, George Mahood. George was recovering from major surgery on his back to fix a condition that could have left him with severe nerve damage. In his hospital bed he motivated himself to do rehab by setting his sights on completing an ironman, and this inspiring and entertaining book chronicles the journey.

- <u>Just a Girl and a Bike: An Unexpected Adventure in Finding Myself</u>, Julie Hiner. Julie falls in love with cycling and pursues it a lot further than most of us- her and her husband climb many iconic routes in Europe made famous by the Tour De France and Giro d'Italia. What may have been most inspiring was their grinding away on bike trainers indoors to stay in shape during Calgary's winters.

- <u>World Class: The Making of the U.S. Women's Cross-Country Ski Team</u>, Peggy Shinn. The amazing story of the US team's rise from obscurity to winning gold at the 2018 Winter Olympics in PyeongChang.

- <u>The Mountains are Calling: Running in the High Places of Scotland</u>, Jonny Muir. A fun chronicle of loving the outdoors and especially fell running, with beautiful descriptions of challenging locations in Scotland.

- <u>Shut Up, Legs!: My Wild Ride On and Off the Bike</u>, Jens Voigt, James D. Startt. "Jensy" (pronounced Yensy) is one of my favorite professional cyclists, with a great sense of humor. I and his many fans loved watching his awesome displays of stamina, winning race stages often with long solo breakaways. His autobiography starts with his youth in East Germany behind the iron curtain and continues through his illustrious career, culminating in him breaking one of cycling's greatest challenges, the hour record.

- <u>Standing Cyclist: Flirting with Wisdom, One Breath, One Mile at a Time</u>, Frank Angelo Cavaluzzi. Frank is a fellow amateur athlete who thinks outside the box. He describes some of his unusual feats like completing a long distance off-road cycle tour on a long wheelbase recumbent, and creating custom bikes on which he does long distance adventures, standing up to pedal. One of these was a fixed gear bike he took on a long challenge in the mountains (without sitting or being able to coast downhill).

- <u>Dividing the Great</u>, John Metcalfe. There are multiple good and inspiring chronicles about cycling the Continental Divide Trail from Canada to Mexico. I found John's to be the most entertaining.

- <u>Old Man on a Bicycle: A Ride Across America and How to Realize a More Enjoyable Old Age</u>, Don Petterson. Don rides his bike across the US after retiring, and this is an enjoyable account of his journey. This sets the bar pretty high for staying active as we age.

- <u>Keep on Moving!: An Old Fellow's Journey into the World of Rollators, Mobile Scooters, Recumbent Trikes, Adult Trikes and Electric Bikes</u>, Allen Ballard. Allen had to give up driving in his 80s due to physical infirmities. This is his search for a way to keep moving. First he describes walking with a rollator (an improved walker design that my Mom used). This is not the shuffle you're used to seeing with a regular walker, but real power walking. Then he describes his odyssey that ends up leading to an electric-assist trike with a very low step-over height, which he now uses to travel all around his neighborhood. If Allen can do this in his late 80s, what excuse do the rest of us have for not moving?

Heart Valve Surgery

- <u>Opening My Heart: A Journey from Nurse to Patient and Back Again</u>, Tilda Shalof. An insider's look at going through heart valve surgery and recovery. Tilda is an experienced nurse so has great insight into the medical system.
- <u>The Patient's Guide To Heart Valve Surgery</u>, Adam Pick. Adam recounts in detail his own open heart surgery, and also gives many tips for other patients who are facing the procedure. Adam also started and maintains the website www.heart-valve-surgery.com. This has a lot of useful information, a surgeon finder, a patient news feed where you can get your questions answered, and success stories from many patients (including yours truly).

Fitness

- <u>Challenge Yourself</u>, Clarence Bass. Clarence has written many good books on fitness. This is my favorite because he motivates us to set challenges to inspire us to work harder. Clarence also has a lot of inspiration and information on nutrition and fitness on his website www.cbass.com.
- <u>The One-Minute Workout: Science Shows a Way to Get Fit That's Smarter, Faster</u>, Dr. Martin Gibala. Based on his pioneering research, Dr. Gibala has come up with a program to achieve fitness benefits with a minimal time investment. The book also has good information on interval training in general.
- <u>The Haywire Heart: How Too Much Exercise Can Kill You, And What You Can Do To Protect Your Heart</u>, Case Christopher J., Mandrola Dr. John, Zinn Lennard. An excellent chronicle of how too much aerobic exercise, especially at moderate intensity, can cause heart problems like atrial fibrillation and other arrhythmias.
- <u>Endure: Mind, Body, and the Curiously Elastic Limits of Human Performance</u>, Alex Hutchinson. A fascinating account of recent knowledge from science and elite athletes on pushing back the limits of fitness.
- <u>No Sweat: How The Simple Science Of Motivation Can Bring You A Lifetime Of Fitness</u>, Dr. Michelle Segar. Techniques for motivating us to work fitness into our lifestyles, from a psychologist who specializes in this.
- <u>Get Up!: Why Your Chair is Killing You and What You Can Do About It</u>, Dr. James Levine. Motivation to keep moving throughout the day by one of the pioneers in the field of non-exercise activity thermogenesis.

- <u>Strength Training Past 50- 3rd Edition</u>, Wayne Westcott, Thomas Baechle. A good introduction to strength training for us older folks.
- <u>Heavyhands Walking</u>, Dr. Leonard Schwartz. A good discussion of Dr. Schwartz's heavyhands technique. As shown in the book, this is a time efficient and enjoyable complete exercise approach.
- <u>Run Forever</u>, Amby Burfoot. Amby was the winner of the Boston Marathon in 1968 and recently completed it in 2018 on the 50th anniversary of his victory. Interesting stories and good tips on running from his lifetime of experience.
- <u>Balance is Power</u>, Jim Klopman. A good discussion of how balance degrades with age, but is readily trainable with a small time commitment. Jim's techniques have worked very well for me.
- <u>The Time-Crunched Cyclist: Race-Winning Fitness in 6 Hours a Week</u>, Carmichael Chris, Rutberg Jim. Famous cycling coach Chris Carmichael shows how to achieve a high level of fitness in a reasonable amount of time that more readily fits into our lifestyle.

Healthy Eating and Weight Loss

- <u>Always Hungry?</u>, Dr. David Ludwig. Dr. Ludwig's breakthrough technique for resetting our metabolisms. A great discussion of how modern processed foods have messed up our metabolisms and how to fix it.
- <u>How Not To Die</u>, Dr. Michael Gregor. Information and inspiration on the health benefits of a whole food plant based diet and how it helps with various "diseases of civilization.

- <u>The Spectrum: How to Customize a Way of Eating and Living Just Right for You and Your Family</u>, Dr. Dean Ornish. Dr Ornish is famous for his program for reversing coronary artery disease that includes a strict wfpb diet. In this book he shows how those of use that are trying to prevent heart disease, not reverse it, can achieve good health results with a looser diet.
- <u>Wired To Eat</u>, Rob Wolf. Rob is an advocate of the paleo diet and has helped thousands of clients with it. He gives fascinating scientific evidence how diet is not one size fits all but is customizable to each individual.
- <u>Mini Habits for Weight Loss</u>, Stephen Guise. A good discussion of why conventional approaches, especially those involving calorie restriction, have a very low success rate. Stephen instead shows how to ease into a healthier lifestyle that will lead to long term weight loss by making small changes that have a cumulative effect.
- <u>Salt Sugar Fat: How the Food Giants Hooked Us</u>, Michael Moss. Fascinating history of the modern processed food industry and discussion of how food science optimizes the addictive power of processed food.
- <u>The Blue Zones Solution: Eating and Living Like the World's Healthiest People</u>, Dan Buettner. Interesting and inspiring discussion of populations around the world that have diets and lifestyle that lead to improved health and longevity.
- <u>Slim by Design: Mindless Eating Solutions for Everyday Life</u>, Dr. Brian Wansink. From an expert in the field of mindless eating, a description of how to change our home environments and habits so that we automatically make better food choices.

Stress Relief and Meditation

- The Relaxation Response, Herbert Benson M.D., Miriam Z. Klipper. A pioneering demystified and scientific description of meditation and its health benefits, with good instruction on meditation. The original version from 1975 has stood the test of time. This updated 2009 edition has interesting new information.
- Mindful Running: How Meditative Running can Improve Performance and Make you a Happier, More Fulfilled Person, Mackenzie L. Havey. A good discussion of how to achieve "meditation in motion" while running, but the techniques discussed can readily be modified for other repetitive activities like walking, cycling, and swimming as well.
- Meditation Is Not What You Think: Mindfulness and Why It Is So Important, Jon Kabat-Zinn. Dr Kabat-Zinn was a pioneer in introducing mindfulness meditation to Western medicine, founding Mindfulness Based Stress Reduction. This book gives his advice on mindfulness and meditation.
- The Miracle of Mindfulness: An Introduction to the Practice of Meditation, Thich Nhat Hanh. The first book I encountered on mindfulness by a Buddhist monk from Vietnam who founded Plum Village in France during the Vietnam war. This is a simple and elegant introduction to mindfulness practice.
- Let Your Mind Run: A Memoir of Thinking My Way to Victory, Deena Kastor, Michelle Hamilton. Olympian Deana Kastor's memoirs of using positive thinking to improve her athletic performance and her life.

Social Support

- <u>Healthy at 100: The Scientifically Proven Secrets of the World's Healthiest and Longest-Lived Peoples</u>, John Robbins. John covers some healthy and long-lived populations like the Okinawans, the Hunzas of Central Asia, and the inhabitants of Vilcabamba in the Andes. He shows the importance of their diet as well as other lifestyle factors, of which social support is vital.
- <u>Love and Survival: Healing Power of Intimacy</u>, Dean Ornish. Dr Ornish shows how intimacy improves our health as well as the quality of our lives. Support groups are an important aspect of his lifestyle programs for good health.

References

1. Aiello L, Wheeler P., "The expensive-tissue hypothesis: The brain and the digestive system in human and primate evolution". Current Anthropology, 1995

2. Bae S., et al, "Plasma choline metabolites and colorectal cancer risk in the Women's Health Initiative Observational Study.", Cancer Res. 2014

3. Balady, G, "Survival of the Fittest- More Evidence", NEJM, 2002

4. Bilsborough S, Mann, N, "A Review of Issues of Dietary Protein Intake in Humans", International Journal of Sport Nutrition and Exercise Metabolism, 2016

5. Bjerregaard P, Young T, Hegele R, "Low incidence of cardiovascular disease among the Inuit—what is the evidence?", Atherosclerosis. 2003

6. Bohlooli S, et al, "The effect of spinach supplementation on exercise-induced oxidative stress.", J Sports Med Phys Fitness., 2015

7. Bollinger, Lance M, and LaFontaine, Tom, "Exercise and Insulin Resistance:, Strength & Conditioning Journal, 2011

8. Boyle, P, et al, "Effect of Purpose in Life on the Relation Between Alzheimer Disease Pathologic Changes on Cognitive Function in Advanced Age", Arch Gen Psychiatry, 2012

9. Broeder, C, et al, "The effects of either high-intensity resistance or endurance training on resting metabolic rate", The American Journal of Clinical Nutrition, 1992

10. Brouwer I, Wanders A, Katan M, "Effect of animal and industrial trans fatty acids on HDL and LDL cholesterol levels in humans—a quantitative review.", PloS One. 2010

11. Brown, J, et al, "The Gut Microbial Endocrine Organ: Bacterially-Derived Signals Driving Cardiometabolic Diseases", Ann Rev Med., 2015

12. Burke, L, et al, "Low carbohydrate, high fat diet impairs exercise economy and negates the performance benefit from intensified training in elite race walkers", The Journal of Physiology, 2016

13. Caciano, S, Inman C, Gockel-Blessing E, Weiss E.,"Effects of dietary Acid load on exercise metabolism and anaerobic exercise performance.",J Sports Sci Med., 2015

14. Campbell W, et al, "Increased energy requirements and changes in body composition with resistance training in older adults.", Am J Clin Nutr., 1994

15. Chaves A, "Vasoprotective endothelial effects of a standardized grape product in humans.",Vascul Pharmacol., 2009

16. Chiba M, et al, "Missing environmental factor in inflammatory bowel disease: diet-associated gut microflora.", Inflamm Bowel Dis., 2011

17. Clarke, R, "Dietary lipids and blood cholesterol: quantitative meta-analysis of metabolic ward studies", BMJ, 1997

18. Cordain, L, et al, "Plant-animal subsistence ratios and macronutrient energy estimations in worldwide hunter-gatherer diet", AJCN, 2000

19. Cordain, L, <u>The Paleo Diet</u>, Wiley, 2002

20. Cox, D et al, "Atherosclerosis impairs flow-mediated dilation of coronary arteries in humans.", Circulation, 1989

21. Crowley, <u>Younger Next Year</u>, Workman Publishing Company, 2007

22. Darmadi-Blackberry, I, et al, "Legumes: the most important dietary predictor of survival in older people of different ethnicities.", Asia Pac J Clin Nutr., 2004

23. de Koning, et al., "Low-Carbohydrate Diet Scores and Risk of Type 2 Diabetes in Men," American Journal of Clinical Nutrition, 2011

24. de Punder, K, Pruimboom, L, "The Dietary Intake of Wheat and other Cereal Grains and Their Role in Inflammation", Nutrients., 2013

25. Deopurkar R, et al, "Differential effects of cream, glucose, and orange juice on inflammation, endotoxin, and the expression of Toll-like receptor-4 and suppressor of cytokine signaling-3.", Diabetes Care., 2010

26. Deschenes, M, et al, "Exercise-Induced Hormonal Changes and Their Effects on Skeletal Muscle Tissue", Sports Med, 1991

27. Diaz, K, et al, "Patterns of Sedentary Behavior and Mortality in U.S. Middle-Aged and Older Adults: A National Cohort Study", Annals of Internal Medicine, 2017

28. Donaghue, K, "Beneficial effects of increasing monounsaturated fat intake in adolescents with type 1 diabetes," Diabetes Research and Clinical Practice, 2000

29. Dunlop, D, "Sedentary time in US older adults associated with disability in activities of daily living independent of physical activity", J Phys Act Health., 2015

30. Eaton S, Konner M, "Paleolithic nutrition. A consideration of its nature and current implications.", N Engl J Med., 1985

31. Eaton, S, Shostak, M, and Konner, M, The Paleolithic Prescription, Harper andRow, 1988

32. Echarte M, Ansorena D, Astiasarán I, "Consequences of microwave heating and frying on the lipid fraction of chicken and beef patties.", J Agric Food Chem., 2003

33. Egger G, Vogels N, Westerterp K, "Estimating historical changes in physical activity levels.", The Medical Journal of Australia, 2001

34. Erickson, K, et al, "Physical activity predicts gray matter volume in late adulthood", Neurology, 2010

35. Erridge C, "The capacity of foodstuffs to induce innate immune activation of human monocytes in vitro is dependent on food content of stimulants of Toll-like receptors 2 and 4.", Br J Nutr., 2011

36. Esposito K, et al, "Effect of a mediterranean-style diet on endothelial dysfunction and markers of vascular inflammation in the metabolic syndrome: a randomized

trial.", JAMA., 2004

37. Esselstyn C, "A way to reverse CAD?", J Fam Pract., 2014

38. Estadella, D, et al, "Lipotoxicity: Effects of Dietary Saturated and Transfatty Acids", Mediators of Inflammation, 2013

39. Estruch, R, et al, "Primary Prevention of Cardiovascular Disease with a Mediterranean Diet", NEJM, 2013

40. Estruch R, Salas-Salvadó J., "Towards an even healthier Mediterranean diet",Nutr Metab Cardiovasc Dis. 2013 -2

41. Exler, J, Lemar, L, Smith, J, "Fat and fatty acid content of selected foods containing trans-fatty acids.", A794, 1996

42. Falk, E "Pathogenesis of Atherosclerosis", Journal of the American College of Cardiology, 2006

43. Falony G, Vieira-Silva S, Raes J.,, "Microbiology Meets Big Data: The Case of Gut Microbiota-Derived Trimethylamine.", Annu Rev Microbiol., 2015

44. Feskanich, , D, et al "Walking and Leisure-Time Activity and Risk of Hip Fracture in Postmenopausal Women", JAMA., 2002

45. Fodor, G, et al, "'Fishing' for the Origins of the 'Eskimos and Heart Disease' Story: Facts or Wishful Thinking?", Canadian Journal of Cardiloogy, 2014

46. Forsythe, C, et al, "Limited Effect of Dietary Saturated Fat on Plasma Saturated Fat in the Context of a Low Carbohydrate Diet", Lipids, 2010

47. Fuhrman, J, Eat to Live, Little, Brown and Company, 2011

48. Fung, T, et al, "Low-Carbohydrate Diets and All-Cause and Cause-Specific Mortality: Two Cohort Studies," Annals of Internal Medicine, 2010

49. Gearhardt A, et al, " The addiction potential of hyperpalatable foods", Current Drug Abuse Reviews, 2011

50. Gibala, M, and Shulgan, C, The One Minute Workout, Avery, 2017

51. Gortner, W, "Nutrition in the United States, 1900 to 1974", Cancer Research, 1975

52.   Graf, E, Eaton, J, "Suppression of colonic cancer by dietary phytic acid", Nutr. Cancer , 1993

53.   Graf, E, Epson, L, Eaton, J "Phytic acid: a natural anitoxidant. J. Biol. Chem, 1987

54.   Greenfield, B, <u>The Low Carb Athlete</u>, Ben Greenfield Fitness, 2015

55.   Gregor, M, Stone, G, <u>How Not to Die</u>, Flatiron Books, 2015

56.   Grivetti, L, "Mediterranean Food Patterns", in The Mediterranean Diet: Constituents and Health Promotion, Matalas, et al, eds, CRC Press, 2001

57.   Groennebaek, T, Vissing, K "Impact of Resistance Training on Skeletal Muscle Mitochondrial Biogenesis, Content, and Function", Front Physiol., 2017

58.   Guimaraes, G, et al, "Effects of continuous vs. interval exercise training on blood pressure and arterial stiffness in treated hypertension", Hypertension Research, 2010

59.   Hamilton, M, et al, "Too Little Exercise and Too Much Sitting: Inactivity Physiology and the Need for New Recommendations on Sedentary Behavior", Curr Cardiovasc Risk Rep., 2008

60.   Hardy, K, et al, "The Importance of Dietary Carbohydrate in Human Evolution", Quarterly Review of Biology, 2015

61.   Harper, R, <u>The Super Carb Diet</u>, St. Martin's Press, 2017

62.   Hartman A, Vining E, Clinical aspects of the ketogenic diet.", Epilepsia., 2007

63.   Hays J, et al, "Effect of a high saturated fat and no-starch diet on serum lipid subfractions in patients with documented atherosclerotic cardiovascular disease.", Mayo Clin Proc., 2003

64.   Heald A, et al, "The influence of dietary intake on the insulin-like growth factor (IGF) system across three ethnic groups: a population-based study.", Public Health Nutr., 2003

65.   Henry, G, et al, "Microfossils in calculus demonstrate consumption of plants and cooked foods in Neanderthal diets (Shanidar III, Iraq; Spy I and II, Belgium)", PNAS, 2011

66.   Hernandez A, et al, "An estimation of the carcinogenic risk associated with the intake of multiple relevant carcinogens found in meat and charcuterie products.", Sci Total Environ., 2015

67.   Hill J, Wyatt H, "Role of physical activity in preventing and treating obesity.",J Appl Physiol (1985)., 2005

68.   Hladik, C, "The human adaptations to meat eating: a reappraisal", Human Evolution, 2002

69.   Hunter, G, et al, "Resistance Training Conserves Fat-free Mass and Resting Energy Expenditure Following Weight Loss", Obesity, 2002

70.   Hunter, G, McCarthy, Bamman, M,"Effects of Resistance Training on Older Adults", Sports Medicine, 2004

71.   Hyman, M, Food: <u>What the Heck Should I Eat?</u>, Little, Brown and Company, 2018

72.   Jensen, et al, "High dietary intake of saturated fat is associated with reduced semen quality among 701 young Danish men from the general population.", Am J Clin Nutr., 2013

73.   Kabat-Zinn, J, <u>Meditation Is Not What You Think: Mindfulness and Why It Is So Important</u>, Hachette Books, 2018

74.   Kateman, Brian, <u>The Reduceitarian Solution</u>, TarcherPerigee, 2017

75.   Katz, M, et al, "Physical Activity Among Amish and Non-Amish Adults Living in Ohio Appalachia", J Community Health, 2012

76.   Kennedy A, et al, "Saturated fatty acid-mediated inflammation and insulin resistance in adipose tissue: mechanisms of action and implications.", J Nutr., 2009

77.   Khor, A, "Postprandial oxidative stress is increased after a phytonutrient-poor food but not after a kilojoule-matched phytonutrient-rich food.",Nutr Res., 2014

78.   Kim M, Hwang SS, Park E, Bae J, "Strict vegetarian diet improves the risk factors associated with metabolic diseases by modulating gut microbiota and reducing intestinal inflammation.", Environ Microbiol Rep., 2013

79.   Lane K, Derbyshire E, Li W, Brennan C, "Bioavailability and potential uses of vegetarian sources of omega-3 fatty acids: a review of the literature.", Crit Rev Food Sci Nutr., 2014

80.   Lee, R, <u>The !Kung San: Men, Women and Work in a Foraging Society</u>, Cambridge University Press, 1979

81.   Lennerz B, et al. "Effects of dietary glycemic index on brain regions related to reward and craving in men", AJCN, 2013

82.   Levine J, "Non-exercise activity thermogenesis (NEAT)", Best Pract Res Clin Endocrinol Metab., 2002

83.   Levine, J, <u>Get Up!: Why Your Chair is Killing You and What You Can Do About It</u>, St. Martin's Press 2014

84.   Li, D, Mehta, J, " Oxidized Ldl, A Critical Factor In Atherogenesis", Cardiovascular Research, 2005

85.   Lindeberg S, et al, "A Palaeolithic diet improves glucose tolerance more than a Mediterranean-like diet in individuals with ischaemic heart disease.", Diabetologia, 2007

86.   Lister, P, et al, "Acacia In Australia: Ethnobotany And Potential Food Crop", In: J. Janick (ed.), Progress in new crops. ASHS Press, 1996

87.   Little, J, et al, "Low-volume high-intensity interval training reduces hyperglycemia and increases muscle mitochondrial capacity in patients with type 2 diabetes", Journal of Applied Physiology, 2011

88.   Longo, V, <u>The Longevity Diet</u>, Avery, 2018

89.   Loomba R, Arora R, "Statin therapy and aortic stenosis: a systematic review of the effects of statin therapy on aortic stenosis", Am J Ther., 2010

90.   Maffetone, P, <u>Training For Endurance</u>, David Barmore Productions, 1996

91.   Mann G,et al "Cardiovascular Disease in the Masai", Journal of atherosclerosis research, 1964

92.   Mann, G, et al, "Atherosclerosis In The Masai", American Journal of Epidemiology, 1972

93.   Markiewicz L, et al, "Diet shapes the ability of human intestinal microbiota to degrade phytate — in vitro studies.", J Appl Microbiol., 2013

94.   Marlowe, F, Berbesque, J, "Tubers as Fallback Foods and Their Impact on Hadza Hunter-Gatherers", American Journal Of Physical Anthropology, 2009

95.   Mavros, Y, et al, "Mediation of Cognitive Function Improvements by Strength Gains After Resistance Training in Older Adults with Mild Cognitive Impairment: Outcomes of the Study of Mental and Resistance Training", Journal of the American Geriatrics Society, 2016

96.   Mayer, F, et al, "The Intensity and Effects of Strength Training in the Elderly", Dtsch Arztebl Int, v108(21), 2011

97.   McDougall J., "Plant foods have a complete amino acid composition". Circulation, 2002

98.   McLaughlin T, et al, , "Is there a simple way to identify insulin-resistant individuals at increased risk of cardiovascular disease?", Am J Cardiol. 2005

99.   Melnik B, "Leucine signaling in the pathogenesis of type 2 diabetes and obesity.", World J Diabetes, 2012

100.   Melnik, B, et al, "The impact of cow's milk-mediated mTORC1-signaling in the initiation and progression of prostate cancer", Nutrition & Metabolism, 2012

101.   Mendelsohn A, Larrick J, "Dietary modification of the microbiome affects risk for cardiovascular disease.", Rejuvenation Res., 2013

102.   Menshikova, E, et al, "Effects of Exercise on Mitochondrial Content and Function in Aging Human Skeletal Muscle", The Journals of Gerontology, 2006

103.   Messina, M, Messina, V, "Exploring the Soyfood Controversy", Nutrition Today, 2013

104.   Michaelsson, K, et al, "Milk intake and risk of mortality and fractures in women and men: cohort studies", BMJ, 2014

105.   Milton, K, "Hunter-gatherer diets- a different perspective",The American Journal of Clinical Nutrition, 2000

106. Min, J, et al, "Monitoring the formation of cholesterol oxidation products in model systems using response surface methodology", Lipids in Health and Disease, 2015

107. Monte, T, Pritikin, I, Pritikin: The Man Who Healed America's Heart, Rodale, 1987

108. Moss, M, Salt Sugar Fat: How the Food Giants Hooked Us, Random House, 2013

109. Murdock G, "Ethnographic atlas: a summary.", Ethnology, 1967

110. Nelson, M, and Wernick, S, Strong Women Stay Slim, Bantam, 1998

111. Nelson, M, et al "Effects of high-intensity strength training on multiple risk factors for osteoporotic fractures", JAMA, 1994

112. O'Keefe, J, Bell, D, "Postprandial Hyperglycemia/Hyperlipidemia (Postprandial Dysmetabolism) Is a Cardiovascular Risk Factor", Am J Card, 2007

113. O'Keefe, J, et al. "Optimal low-density lipoprotein is 50 to 70 mg/dl Lower is better and physiologically normal", Journal of the American College of Cardiology, 2004

114. Orlich, M, et al, "Vegetarian Dietary Patterns and Mortality in Adventist Health Study 2", JAMA Intern Med., 2013

115. Ornish, D, "Can lifestyle changes reverse coronary heart disease?: The Lifestyle Heart Trial", The Lancet,, 1990

116. Ornish, D, Eat More Weigh Less, William Morrow, 2000.

117. Paffenbarger, R, et al, "Physical Activity, All-Cause Mortality, and Longevity of College Alumni", Nejm, 1986

118. Patterson, E, et al, "Health Implications of High Dietary Omega-6 Polyunsaturated Fatty Acids", J Nutr Metab., 2012

119. Pedrosa, M, et al, "Effects of industrial canning on the proximate composition, bioactive compounds contents and nutritional profile of two Spanish common dry beans (Phaseolus vulgaris L.)", Food Chemistry, 2015

120. Perry, G, et al, ,"Diet and the evolution of human amylase gene copy number variation",Nature Genetics, 2007

121. Phinney, S, Volek, J, <u>The Art and Science of Low Carbohydrate Living</u>, Beyond Obesity LLC, 2011

122. Pick , A, <u>The Patient's Guide To Heart Valve Surgery</u>, Self-published; Revised edition, 2006

123. Pohle, K, et al, "Progression of Aortic Valve Calcification",Circulation, 2001

124. Price, C, <u>How to Break Up with Your Phone</u>, Ten Speed Press, 2018

125. Prior, I, et al, "Cholesterol, coconuts, and diet on Polynesian atolls: a natural experiment: the Pukapuka and Tokelau island studies.", Am J Clin Nutr., 1981

126. Raboy, V, "Progress in Breeding Low Phytate Crops", The Journal of Nutrition, 2002

127. Rainey, I, <u>Still Not Bionic: Adventures In Unremarkable Ultrarunning</u>,Tangent Books, 2016

128. Amitha S, "Kidney Stones and the Ketogenic Diet: Risk Factors and Prevention", Journal of Child Neurology, 2007

129. Ravussin, E, et al, "Effects of a Traditional Lifestyle on Obesity in Pima Indians", Diabetes Care, 1994

130. Reddy, S, et al, editors. <u>Food Phytate</u>, CRC Press, 2002

131. Remer, T, Manz, F, "Potential Renal Acid Load of Foods and its Influence on Urine pH", J Am Diet Assoc., 1995

132. Robbins, J, <u>Healthy at 100: The Scientifically Proven Secrets of the World's Healthiest and Longest-Lived Peoples</u>, Ballantine Books, 2008

133. Sakakibara S, et al, "Vinegar intake enhances flow-mediated vasodilatation via upregulation of endothelial nitric oxide synthase activity.",. Biosci Biotechnol Biochem., 2010

134. Sales-Campos H, et al, "An overview of the modulatory effects of oleic acid in health and disease.", Mini Rev Med Chem., 2013

135. Folan, L, Lilias! <u>Yoga: Your Guide to Enhancing Body, Mind, and Spirit in Midlife and Beyond</u>, Skyhorse

Publishing, 2011

136.   Schofield, G, Zinn, C, Rodgers, C, <u>What the Fat?</u>, The
        Real Food Publishing Company, 2015
137.   Schofield, G, Zinn, C, Rodgers, C, <u>What the Fast?</u>,
        Blackwell and Ruth, 2018
138.   Schwartz, L, <u>Heavyhands Walking Book</u>, Panaerobics
        Press, 1990
139.   Segar, M, <u>No Sweat: How The Simple Science Of
        Motivation Can Bring You A Lifetime Of Fitness</u>,
        HarperCollins, 2015
140.   Shalof, T, <u>Opening My Heart: A Journey from Nurse to
        Patient and Back Again</u>, McClelland & Stewart, 2011
141.   Sharkey, <u>Fitness and Health</u>, 2001
142.   Shephard, R, <u>Aging, Physical Activity, and Health</u>,
        Human Kinetics, 1997
143.   Shintani, T, et al, "Obesity and cardiovascular risk
        intervention through the ad libitum feeding of
        traditional Hawaiian diet", Nutrition, 1991
144.   Shintani, Terry, <u>The Good Carbohydrate Revolution</u>,
        Atria, 2002
145.   Song, J, et, al, "Analysis of Trans Fat in Edible Oils with
        Cooking Process", Toxicol Res., 2015
146.   Song, M, et al, "Association of Animal and Plant Protein
        Intake With All-Cause and Cause-Specific Mortality,"
        JAMA Internal Medicine, 2016
147.   Spiriduso, <u>Physical Dimensions of Aging</u>, Human
        Kinetics, 1995
148.   Stellingwerff, T, et al, "Decreased PDH activation and
        glycogenolysis during exercise following fat adaptation
        with carbohydrate restoration.", Am J Physiol
        Endocrinol Metab., 2006
149.   Storen, O, et al. "The Effect of Age on the VO2max
        Response to High-Intensity Interval Training", Medicine
        & Science in Sports & Exercise, 2017
150.   Tang, W, Hazen S, "The contributory role of gut
        microbiota in cardiovascular disease.", J Clin Invest.,
        2014
151.   Tilg, H, Moschen, A, "Microbiota and diabetes: an
        evolving relationship.", Gut, 2014

152. Tuohy, K, Fava, F, Viola, R, "'The way to a man's heart is through his gut microbiota' — dietary pro- and prebiotics for the management of cardiovascular risk.", Proc Nutr Soc., 2014

153. van den Broeck, H, et al, "Presence of celiac disease epitopes in modern and old hexaploid wheat varieties: wheat breeding may have contributed to increased prevalence of celiac disease.", Theor Appl Genet., 2010

154. van der Ploeg, H, "Sitting time and all-cause mortality risk in 222 497 Australian adults", Arch Intern Med., 2012

155. Venter F, Thiel P., "Red kidney beans — to eat or not to eat?", S Afr Med J. ,1995

156. Vogel, R "Brachial Artery Ultrasound: A Noninvasive Tool in the Assessment of Triglyceride-Rich Lipoproteins",Clin. Cardiol., 1999

157. Volek, J, et, al, "Comparison of energy-restricted very low-carbohydrate and low-fat diets on weight loss and body composition in overweight men and women", Nutr Metab (Lond)., 2004

158. Walker, A, "Are health and ill-health lessons from hunter-gatherers currently relevant?", AJCN, 2001

159. Wang, X, Proud C, "Nutrient control of TORC1, a cell-cycle regulator", Trends Cell Biol., 2009

160. Werner, H, Bruchim, I, "The insulin-like growth factor-I receptor as an oncogene", Arch Physiol Biochem., 2009

161. Willcox, B, et al. "Caloric Restriction, the Traditional Okinawan Diet, and Healthy Aging," Annals of the New York Academy of Science, 2007

162. Williams, J, <u>Slow Fat Triathlete: Live Your Athletic Dreams in the Body You Have Now</u>, Da Capo Lifelong Books, 2004

163. Wolf, R, <u>Wired To Eat</u>, Harmony, 2017

164. Wolk, A, et al, "A Prospective Study of Association of Monounsaturated Fat and Other Types of Fat With Risk of Breast Cancer," Archives of Internal Medicine, 1998

165. Wrangham, R, <u>Catching Fire: How Cooking Made Us Human</u>, Basic Books, 2009

166. Wylde, S, <u>Moving Stretch: Work Your Fascia to Free</u>

Your Body, Penguin,, 2017

167. Zimmerman, M, "The Paleopathology Of The Cardiovascular System",Tex Heart Inst J., 1993

168. www.eatsleep.fit/endurance-sports/fat-burning-why-its-overrated-for-the-competitive-endurance-athlete/

169. www.eatthismuch.com/food/view/white-button-mushrooms-packaged,89993/

170. www.healthline.com/health/food-nutrition/19-high-protein-vegetables

171. www.healthline.com/nutrition/atkins-diet-101

172. http://en.wikipedia.org/wiki/Pedometer

173. www.ers.usda.gov/amber-waves/2010/march/guess-who-s-turning-100tracking-a-century-of-american-eating

174. www.cnpp.usda.gov/sites/default/files/usda_food_patterns/EstimatedCalorieNeedsPerDayTable.pdf

175. Neal C, et al, "Six weeks of a polarized training-intensity distribution leads to greater physiological and performance adaptations than a threshold model in trained cyclists", J Appl Physiol, 2013

176. https://en.wikipedia.org/wiki/Pemmican

177. Zuk, M, Paleofantasy: What Evolution Really Tells Us about Sex, Diet, and How We Live, W. W. Norton & Company, 2014

178. Buettner, D, The Blue Zones: 9 Lessons for Living Longer From the People Who've Lived the Longest, National Geographic, 2012

179. Ludwig, D, Always Hungry?: Conquer Cravings, Retrain Your Fat Cells, and Lose Weight Permanently, Grand Central Life & Style, 2016

180. Spreadbury, I, "Comparison with ancestral diets suggests dense acellular carbohydrates promote an inflammatory microbiota, and may be the primary dietary cause of leptin resistance and obesity", Diabetes Metab Syndr Obes., 2012

181. Schulz, L, Chaudhari, L, "High-Risk Populations: The Pimas of Arizona and Mexico", Curr Obes Rep., 2015

182. Eyres, L, et al, "Coconut oil consumption and

cardiovascular risk factors in humans", Nutrition Reviews, 2016

183. de Lorgeril M, et al, "Mediterranean alpha-linolenic acid-rich diet in secondary prevention of coronary heart disease", Lancet, 1994

184. McDougall J, <u>The Healthiest Diet on the Planet</u>, HarperOne, 2016

185. http://en.wikipedia.org/wiki/Anaerobic_glycolysis

186. http://en.wikipedia.org/wiki/Overtraining

187. http://en.wikipedia.org/wiki/Glycemic_index

188. http://en.wikipedia.org/wiki/FODMAP

189. http://en.wikipedia.org/wiki/Ketogenic_diet#History

190. www.texasheart.org/heart-health/heart-information-center/topics/maze-surgery/

191. www.ted.com/talks/mick_cornett_how_an_obese_town_lost_a_million_pounds

192. American College Of Sports Medicine, "The recommended quantity and quality of exercise for developing and maintaining cardiorespiratory and muscular fitness and flexibility in healthy adults", Med. Sci. Sports Exerc, 1998

193. Ludwig, D, "<u>Always Hungry?</u>", Grand Central Life & Style, 2016

194. Guyenet, S, <u>The Hungry Brain: Outsmarting the Instincts That Make Us Overeat</u>, Flatiron Books, 2017

195. Fumiento, M, <u>Fat of the Land</u>, Penguin, 1997

196. Klopman, J, Miller, J, <u>Balance is Power: Improve Your Body's Balance to Perform Better, Live Longer, and Look Younger</u>, Lioncrest Publishing, 2016

197. Amen, D, <u>The Brain Warrior's Way</u>, Berkley, 2016

198. http://en.wikipedia.org/wiki/Wolff%27s_law

199. Donnison, C, "Blood Pressure In The African Native. Its Bearing Upon The Aetiology Of Hyperptesia And Arterio-sclerosis", The Lancet, 1929

200. Hurd, R, and Hurd, F, <u>Ten Talents Cookbook</u> , published by Dr. Frank J. and Rosalie Hurd; Improved edition, April 2, 2012

201.   Anderson, O, <u>Running Science</u>, Human Kinetics, 2013

202.   Tabata, I, et al, "Effects Of Moderate-intensity Endurance Training And High-intensity Intermittent Training On Anaerobic Capacity And VO2max", Medicine and Science in Sport and Exercise, 1997

203.   Esselstyn, C, <u>Prevent and Reverse Heart Disease: The Revolutionary, Scientifically Proven, Nutrition-Based Cure</u>, Avery, 2007

204.   http://www.johnmuirhealth.com/services/cardiovascular-services/intervention/transcatheter-aortic-valve-replacement/facts-and-figures.html

205.   Adlercreutz, H, "Phytoestrogens and Breast Cancer", The Journal of Steroid Biochemistry and Molecular Biology, 2002

206.   Franceschi, C, et al, "Inflamm-aging: An Evolutionary Perspective on Immunosenescence", Annals of the New York Academy of Sciences, 2016

207.   Kastor, D, <u>Let Your Mind Run</u>, Crown Archetype, 2018

208.   Benson, H, Klipper, M, <u>The Relaxation Response</u>, HarperCollins, 2009

209.   www.runnersworld.com/nutrition-weight-loss/a20856840/eat-like-an-elite-jim-walmsley/

210.   Morton, M, et al, "The Complete Health Improvement Program (CHIP)", American Journal of Lifestyle Medicine, 2014

211.   Kossoff, E, "Danger in the Pipeline for the Ketogenic Diet?", Epilepsy Curr., 2014

212.   Best T, et al, "Cardiac complications in pediatric patients on the ketogenic diet", Neurology., 2000

213.   Barclay G, et al, "The effect of dietary yeast on the activity of stable chronic Crohn's disease", Scand J Gastroenterol, 1992

214.   Chiba, M, et al, "Plant-Based Diets in Crohn's Disease", Perm J., 2014

215.   Pollock, R, et al, "Properties of the vastus lateralis muscle in relation to age and physiological function in master cyclists aged 55-79 years", Aging Cell., 2018

216.   Duggal, N, et al, "Major features of immunesenescence, including reduced thymic output, are ameliorated by

high levels of physical activity in adulthood", Aging Cell, 2018

217. Rothschild , J, and Earnest, C, "Dietary Manipulations Concurrent to Endurance Training", J. Funct. Morphol. Kinesiol., 2018

218. Seiler KS, Kjerland G, "Quantifying training intensity distribution in elite endurance athletes: is there evidence for an "optimal" distribution?", Scand J Med Sci Sports., 2006

219. Fardet, A. "Minimally processed foods are more satiating and less hyperglycemic than ultra-processed foods: A preliminary study with 98 ready-to-eat foods" , Food Funct, 2016

220. King, A., et al, "Behavioral impacts of sequentially versus simultaneously delivered dietary plus physical activity interventions: the CALM Trial", Annals of Behavioral Medicine, 2013

221. Coyle, E, "Very Intense Exercise-Training Is Extremely Potent and Time Efficient: A Reminder." J Appl Physiol., 2005

222. Burgomaster, K, et al, "Six sessions of sprint interval training increases muscle oxidative potential and cycle endurance capacity in humans", J Appl Phys, 2005

223. Melov, S, et al, "Resistance Exercise Reverses Aging in Human Skeletal Muscle", Plos One, 2007

224. Gilligan, L, et al, "Aerobic Interval Training vs. Continuous Moderate Exercise in the Metabolic Syndrome of Rats Artificially Selected for Low Aerobic Capacity." Cardiovasc Res, 2009

225. Babraj J, et al "Extremely short duration high intensity interval training substantially improves insulin action in young healthy males", BMC Endocr, 2009

226. Gaesser, G and Weltman, A, "Effect of Exercise Training Intensity on Abdominal Visceral Fat and Body Composition", Med Sci Sports Exer, 2008

227. Chakravarthy, M, and Booth, F, "Eating, exercise, and 'thrifty' genotypes: connecting the dots toward an evolutionary understanding of modern chronic diseases", J Appl Phys, 2003

228. Lee, I, et al;. "Relative Intensity of Physical Activity and Risk of Coronary Heart Disease." Circulation, 2003

229. Bruce C, et al, "Muscle oxidative capacity is a better predictor of insulin sensitivity than lipid status", J Clin Endocrinol Metab., 2003

230. López-González A, et al, "Phytate (myo-inositol hexaphosphate) and risk factors for osteoporosis", J Med Food., 2008

231. López-González A, et al, "Protective effect of myo-inositol hexaphosphate (phytate) on bone mass loss in postmenopausal women", Eur J Nutr., 2013

232. Devore E, et al, "Dietary intakes of berries and flavonoids in relation to cognitive decline", Ann Neurol., 2012

233. O'Brien J, et al, "Long-term intake of nuts in relation to cognitive function in older women.", J Nutr Health Aging, 2014

234. Tuttle, K, "The 'Eco-Atkins' Diet, New Twist on an Old Tale", JAMA, 2018

235. Sadik-Khan, J, and Solomonow, S, <u>Streetfight: Handbook for an Urban Revolution</u>, Penguin Books, 2016

www.ingramcontent.com/pod-product-compliance
Lightning Source LLC
Chambersburg PA
CBHW031054250726

48655CB00004B/1430